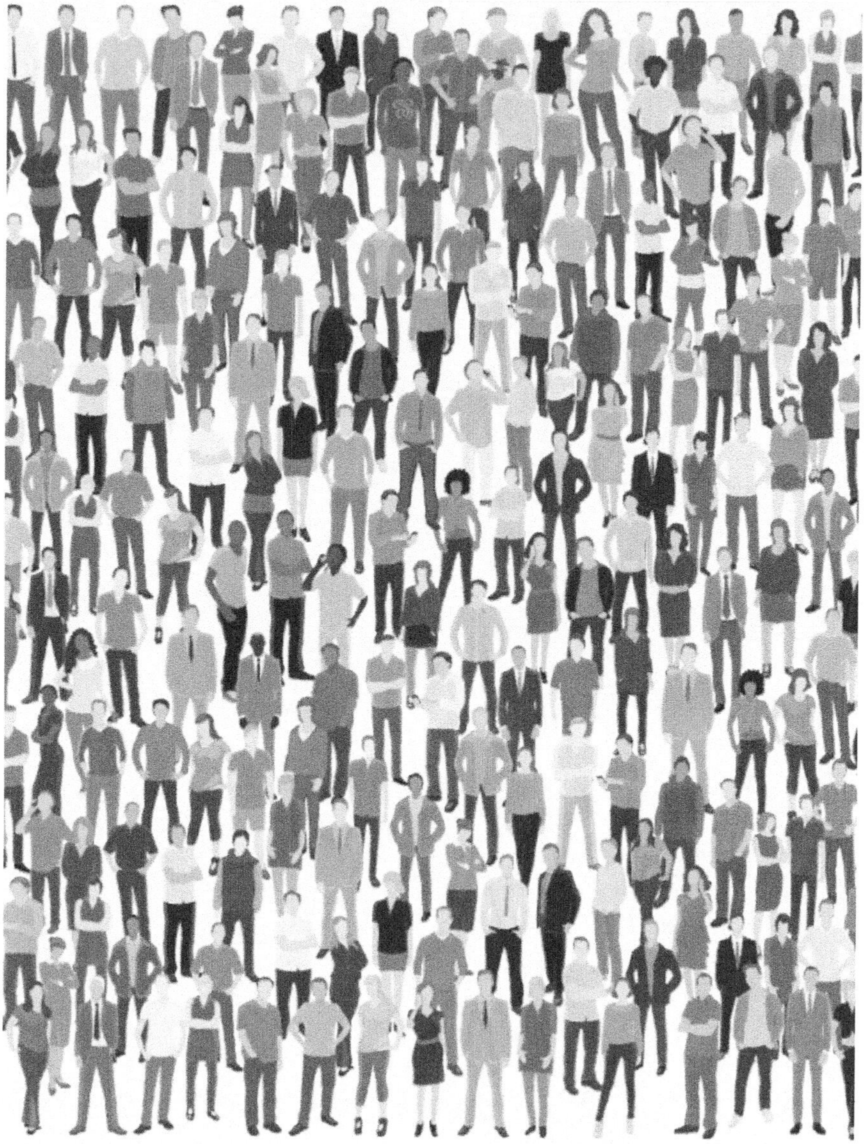

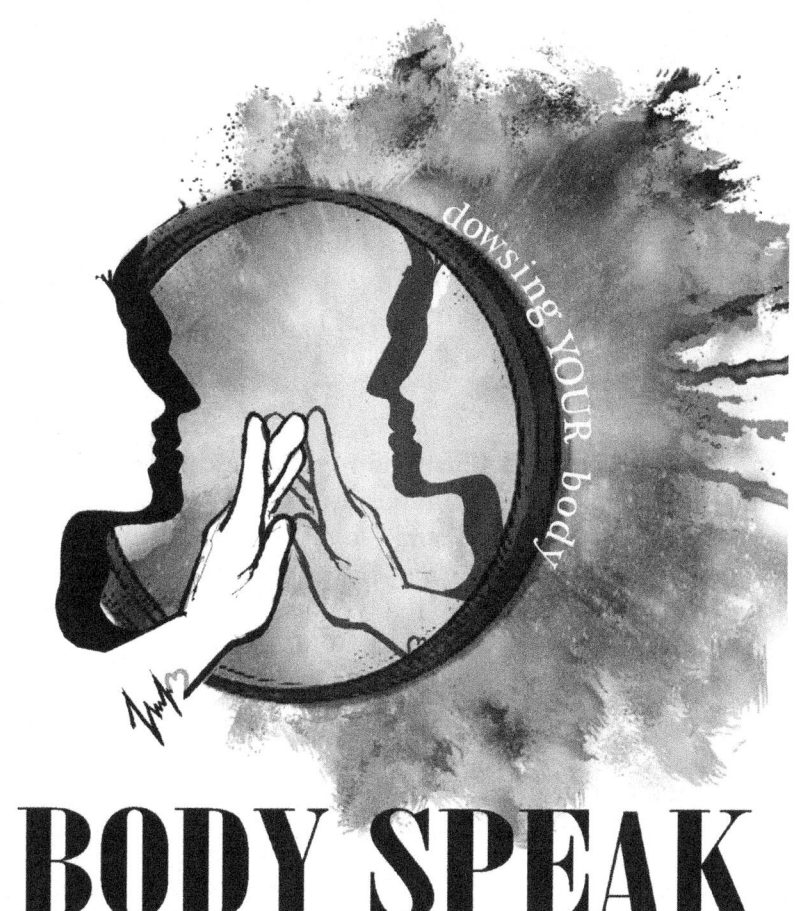

BODY SPEAK

by Isabell VanMerlin

BODY SPEAK**, Revised Second Edition**
Cover image by Lenka Lesnak McDonald
      https://www.facebook.com/MebyLenka/
      https://www.instagram.com/mebylenka/?hl=en
Author photo by Nicoletta Camerin
      https://www.nikiphotographysonoma.com/

Photographs and illustrations by Isabell VanMerlin,
    with great thanks to Dr. James Peck (DC), and Dr. Audrey Peck (DC), for being my willing and photogenic models.

Copyright © 2020, Isabell VanMerlin, Dover, NH 03820

First edition photo and illustration credits are owed to: Peggy Koenig, Marian Sinclair, and author, Ana Belle Whiting, nka Isabell VanMerlin. Larry Gillespie and Donna Westing were wonderful and wonderfully photogenic models; and thanks also go to Bob, artist model, of The Drawing Studio of Tucson.
    Copyright © 1999 Ana Belle Whiting
    Published by **Peggy's Prints**
    Tucson, Arizona 85705

PLEASE BE ADVISED: I am not a medical doctor; I am not a licensed health professional of any kind. The dowsing techniques and alternative therapies presented in this book are for people who are interested in health, preventative and alternative therapies, and are willing to take responsibility for their own health. The examples are my own experiences and the therapies and techniques are suggestions. I can offer no guarantees and therefore can accept no liability. I do sincerely hope that some of you will be encouraged by this book in your search for better health and in finding answers to your questions.

Dedicated to my teacher Sarah Meredith,
wherever she may be,
and my mother,
who got me interested in all this,
despite my best resistance.

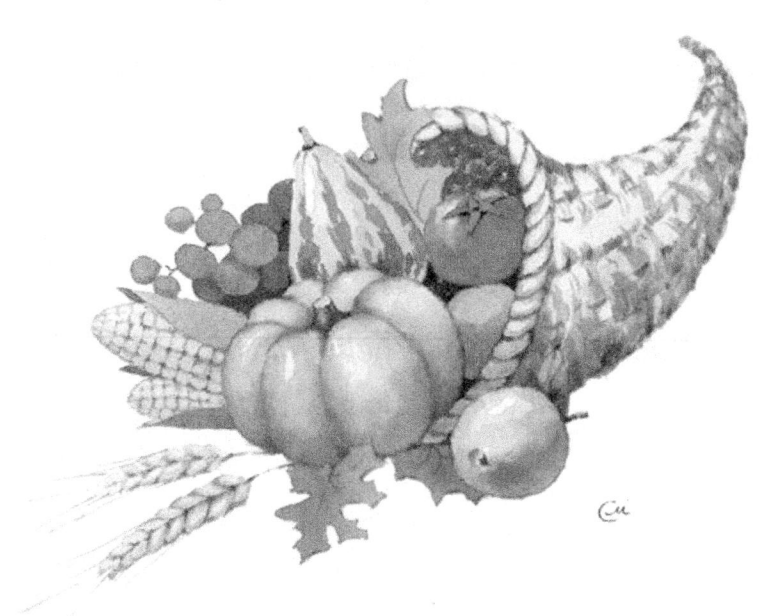

Contents

ACKNOWLEDGMENTS i
APOLOGY iii
INTRODUCTION vii
SPECIAL NOTE ON SELF DOWSING xvii
  1. THE BASICS 1
      A.   MUSCLE TESTING 1
      B.   INTENTION: ROOT CAUSE 11
      C.   PERMISSION? 15
      D.   POWER ON? 23
  2. PRIMARY PHYSICAL POINTS 33
  3. SECONDARY PHYSICAL POINTS 91
  4. REMEDIES 133
  5. BLOOD TYPE DIET 143
  6. NEURO-EMOTIONAL RELEASING 153
  7. SPIRITUAL RESPONSE THERAPY 163
  8. NEW THOUGHT 167

BIBLIOGRAPHY 173

Thank you

Thanks, ahéhee' (Navajo), arigato gozaimasu (ありがとうございます Japanese), asante (Swahili), blagodarya (благодаря Bulgarian), ďakujem (Slovak), děkuji (Czech), danke (German), dankon (Esperanto), dhanwaad (ਧੰਨਵਾਦ Punjabi), dhanyawad (धन्यवाद Hindi), diolch (Welsh), dziękuję (Polish), e sé (Yoruba), efharisto (ευχαριστώ Greek), gracias (Spanish), gratias tibi ago (Latin), grazie (Italian), köszönöm (Hungarian), khawp khun (ขอบคุณ Thai), mahalo (Hawaiian), merci (French), mulțumesc (Romanian), nandri (நன்றி Tamil), obrigado (Portuguese), salamat (Tagalog), shnorhakalutyoon (Շնորհակալություն Armenian), shukran (شكرا Arabic), spasibo (Спасибо Russian), takk (Faroese), takk (Icelandic), teşekkür ederim (Turkish), toda (תודה Hebrew), xièxie(謝謝 Chinese traditional, 谢谢 simplified), ...

(A FEW)
ACKNOWLEDGMENTS

I want to particularly thank Gail Johnson, a Texas dowser, massage therapist and loving human being for saying to me, "Haven't you written a book on this?" or some such similar words on April 14, 1998. That was what I needed to get serious about putting this book together.

My dear, wonderful, smart, creative and supportive friend Peggy Koenig saw me through yet another of my "projects," and her desktop publishing expertise and savvy greatly enhanced the quality of the first edition of this book not to mention making it manifest in physical, literary form.

Mary Abdoo, Deepak Chopra, Wayne Dyer, Marianne Williamson, Rev. Rainbow Johnson, Sandra Musser, Monroe Rust, Dr. King, Jackie Dennis, Rhea Loudon, Mr. A., Kari Cannistraro, Aunty Caroline and Uncle Walter are but a few of the teachers that have made such a difference to me and without whose relationships my life, and this book, would have been boring way beyond words.

BODY SPEAK

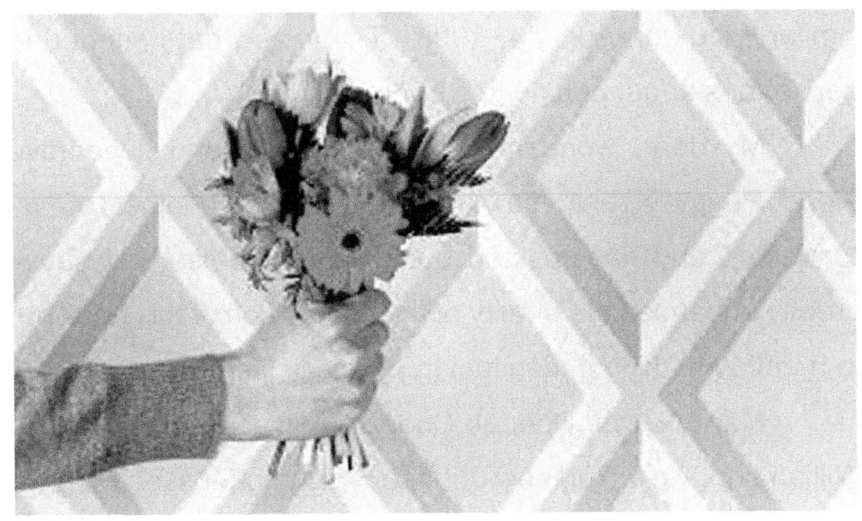

APOLOGY

I have to tell you right now, before you go any further, that I probably should not be putting this book into print again. Things have changed so drastically in the world: technology, medicine – and in MY life since I first wrote *Body Speak* that I feel something of a piker or a charlatan in presenting this. I have come to believe that our bodies, and our physical, material world are not REAL in any permanent sense – but that only SPIRIT is REAL (capital letters) - even though everything is made of Spirit, including our physical, material world. I believe we have been created from Divine Mind; that we are expressions of Divine Mind. And that we are PERFECT. I believe we are here on this planet to REALIZE our perfection because somehow we have forgotten that we are part of God / Divine Mind / Cosmic Consciousness, that we are perfect, and are loved unconditionally.

Of course I have an earthsuit, as we all do, but I don't want to buy into the appearance of 'problems' – physical problems, health problems, *any* problems. At the same time,

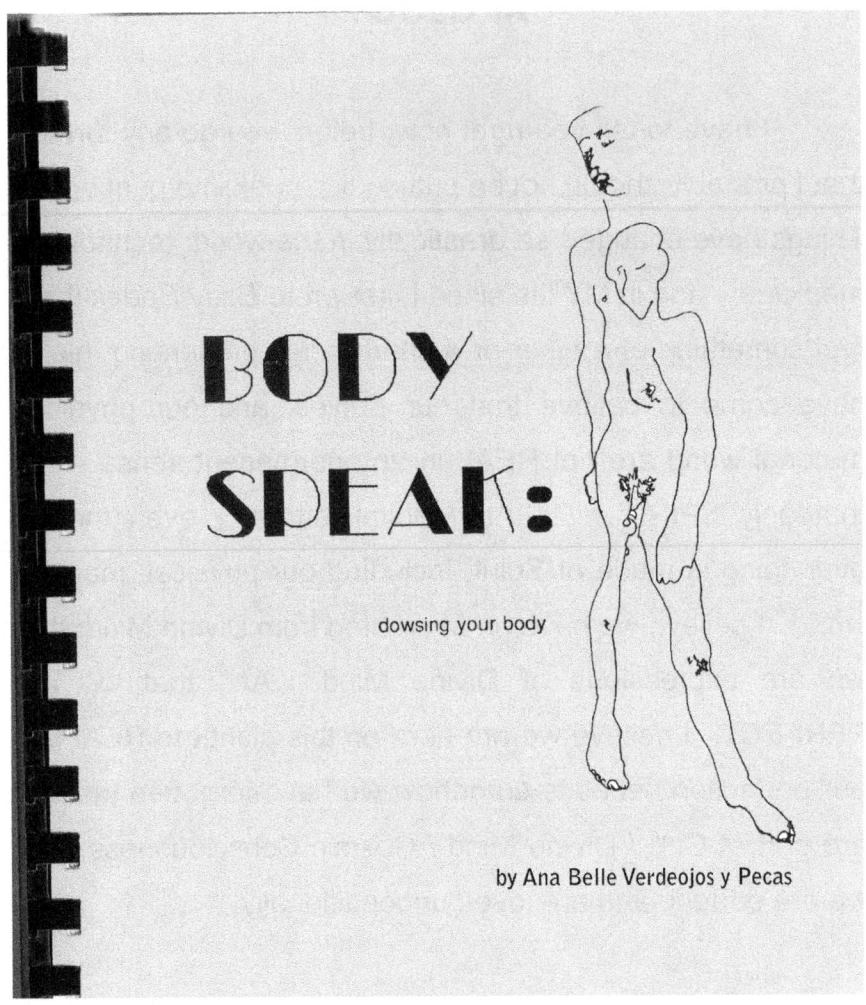

This was the original cover of Body Speak
and I owe Bob, from The Drawing Studio,
an apology for what my awkward pen did to his body.
I hope he never knows . . . please don't tell him!

our bodies are the sacred temples of Spirit, and we're here on earth living in these physical bodies. And we are here to learn.

So, what is the answer?

The conclusion I have come to is that we must keep working on our spirituality while caring for our earthsuits! While I don't use all these therapies all the time now, my intention is to make the knowledge I have acquired over the years available to others. Use what works for you and leave the rest. The most important thing is to KNOW that YOU are PERFECT and LOVED UNCONDITIONALLY!

BODY SPEAK

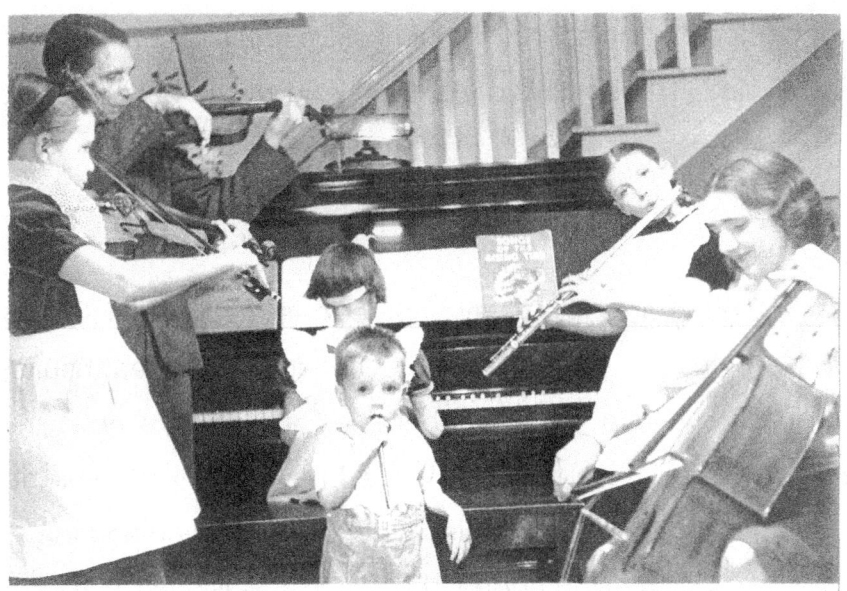

Mother said I cried when I saw this picture and was not in it; she tried to explain to me I wasn't born yet!

INTRODUCTION

    Several years before I was conceived, much less born, my mother acquired a tumor on one ovary. She was already very interested in health foods and nutrition and she searched out a naturopath or osteopath not too far from us, in North Carolina, who was a student of Max Gerson[1]. After only a couple of months drinking raw vegetable juices and eating steamed greens (primarily), having coffee enemas and gradually adding small amounts of yogurt to her very strict diet, the tumor completely disappeared! I believe that I was the recipient of the "best" of her genes, even though I was the fifth and youngest child of the family, because of this cleansing and healing program that she followed. (This rejuvenation program did not produce the desired second son, however!)

    As the years went by after I was born, my mother continued her studies of nutrition and health foods, subscribing to *Prevention* magazine and reading all of Adelle

---

[1] Max Gerson, M.D., was a contemporary of Sigmund Freud, who also hailed from Vienna. He developed a very effective, primarily nutritional therapy for cancer. His daughter Charlotte continues to heal using her father's cancer therapy at The Gerson Institute in San Diego, CA.

BODY SPEAK

Tell me what you eat, and I will tell you what you are.

> Anthelme Brillat-Savaarin
> [1755-1826]
> *La Physiologie du Gout*, "Fundamental Truths"
> (tr. By R.E. Anderson as *Gastronomy as a Fine Art*)

You are what you eat.

> American Proverb
> Since 1941

INTRODUCTION

Davis' books. My brother and I strenuously objected to her homemade whole wheat bread and carrot juice when we were teenagers. I'll never forget the occasion when my brother asked her, "How are cinder blocks made, Mother? And how much do you think they cost to make?"

After Mother gave him her best, most serious guesstimate, my brother came forth with,

"Well, how much does it cost you to make your bread?"

She came close to braining him with a cast iron skillet!

Rebellion for me took the form of going to the next-door neighbors' and drinking soft drinks with my friend at every possible opportunity; they bought pop by the case whereas Mother never allowed it in our house. Even in the 50's my mother knew that soda was worse than 'no-count' for your health, phosphoric acid destroying calcium and carbonated water disturbing the stasis of your cells which, in turn, allows germs and/or viruses to penetrate the cell walls and create infections when the walls are weakend.

My mother DID love "brown cows" (vanilla ice cream in root beer), however, and would order one as a treat when we went out. I realized much later that my mother had quite

BODY SPEAK

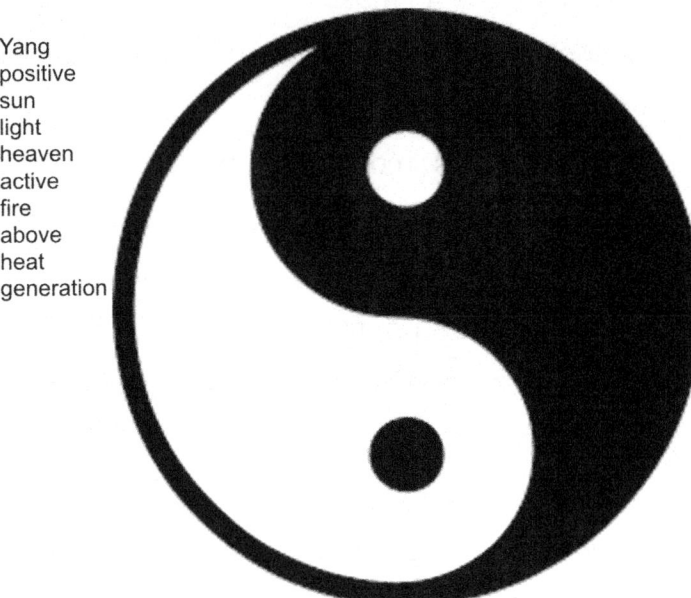

Yang
positive
sun
light
heaven
active
fire
above
heat
generation

Yin
negative
moon
dark
earth
passive
water
below
cold
growth

INTRODUCTION

a terrible sweet tooth, and I guess she tried to make her family eat healthfully in order to assuage her own conscience: a "Do as I say, not (necessarily) as I do" attitude.

Dowsing is a "polarized" tool. We live on a polarized planet that has north and south poles at the opposite ends of the earth. This polarization perhaps explains our penchant for wanting to make things positive or negative, light or dark, good or evil – safe or scary. Our evolution, however, is taking us to a place of balance. Instead of reliance on an immune system to DEFEND our bodies, we are moving towards a BALANCE that makes defense unnecessary for good health. This balance is controlled, or perhaps better said, managed in our bodies through the endocrine system. The endocrine system is the system of glands and organs that are the autonomic nervous system (heart pump, digestion, menstrual cycle, etc.). Listening to our bodies speak, we can consciously help not only the autonomic nervous system, but our endocrine system and every other part and function of our bodies to maintain balance and health.

Western Medicine uses medicine/drugs to treat *symptoms* of illness and dis-ease. Ayurveda ("knowledge of

BODY SPEAK

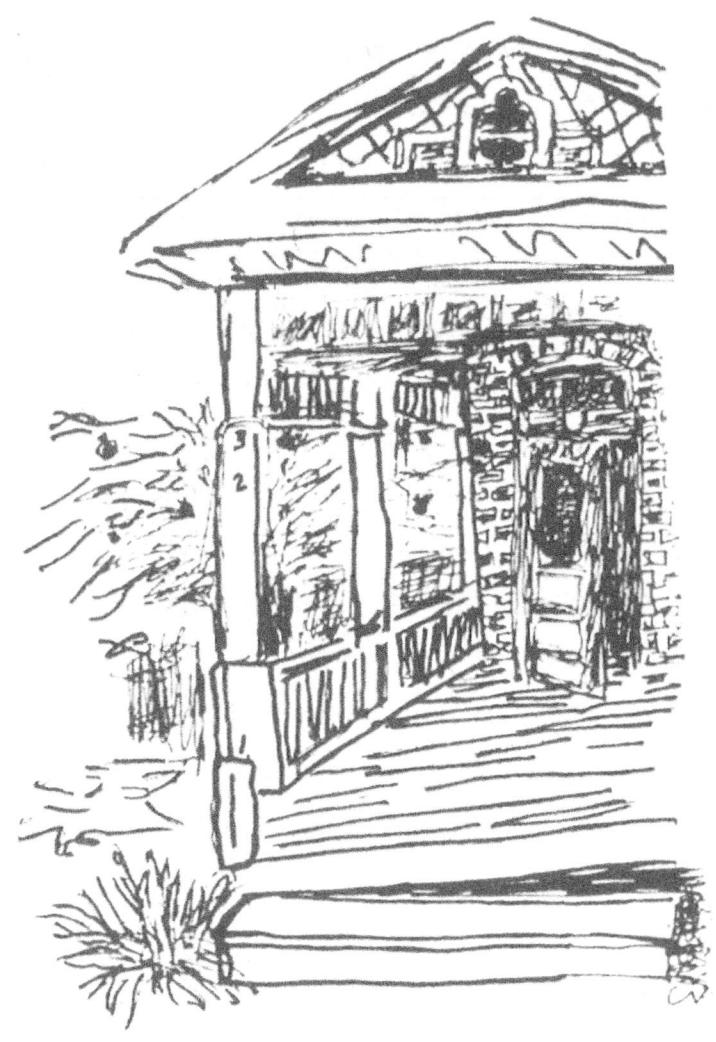

East 17th Street, Tucson
home of the first edition

INTRODUCTION

life and longevity") is an ancient healing practice that comes from the Indian subcontinent and uses herbal compounds, minerals and metal substances for restoring balance to the body. Chinese acupuncture is used mainly for pain relief, but also to restore energy balance to the "hot spots," the places that are causing pain or are infirm. In Body Speak, we use some of the acupuncture or acupressure points of the various glands and organs of our bodies in order to find the malfunctioning places – and then, hopefully, to heal the offending part!

No matter what our path or perspective, we are all here to heal and to integrate body, mind and spirit. We are also here to share our talents, i.e., BE WHO WE ARE, i.e., EXPRESS OURSELVES. This is my contribution, be what it may, to the Universal Process and the Cosmic Consciousness, of which WE ARE ALL ONE. I AM grateful.

Ana Belle Verdeojos y Pecas
(*green eyes and freckles*)
Tucson, Arizona
December 6, 1998

BODY SPEAK

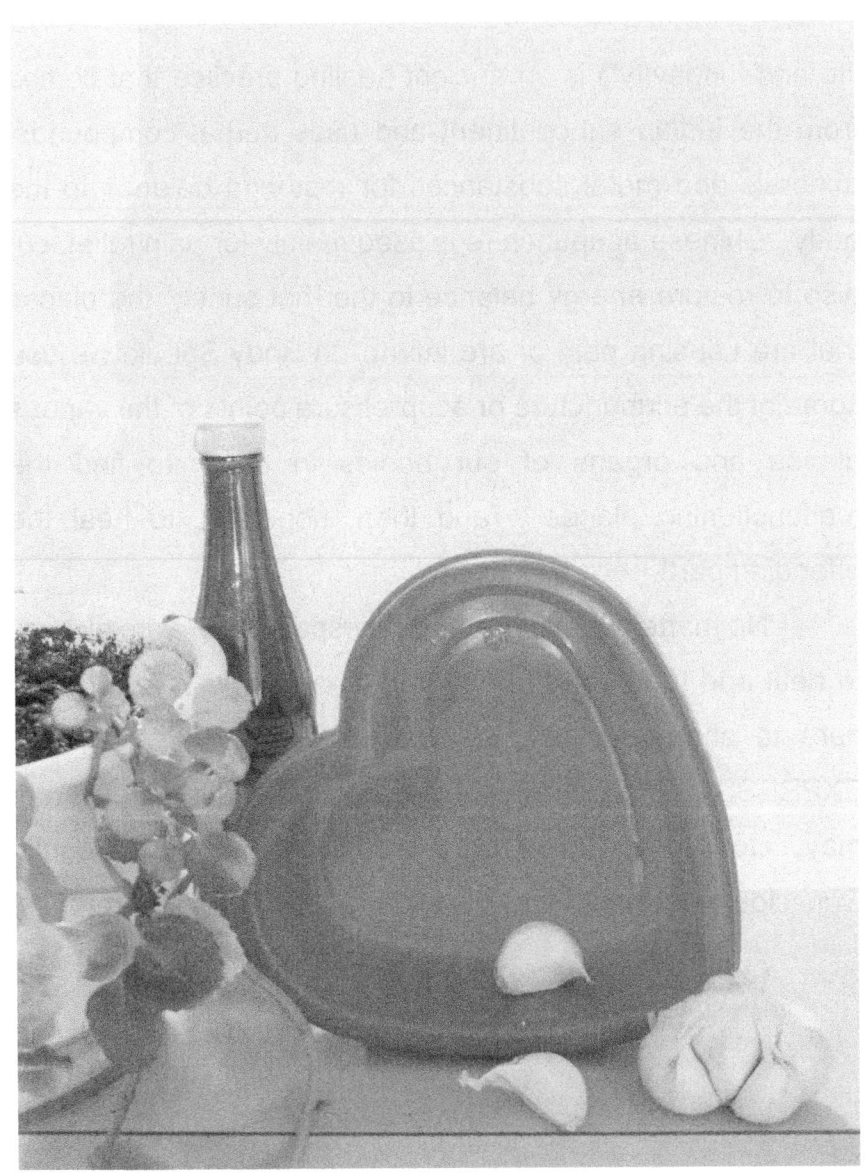

INTRODUCTION

I never had an electronic copy of my book when I first wrote it – back in the digital dark ages. Twenty years have gone by (holy smokes!) and I have found a few changes and errors, and needed to update other things. I also have had some wonderful experiences since then. So here is Edition 2.

One of the changes is a section on the nutritional therapy *Eat Right 4 Your Type* (blood type), a major discovery for me – one that everyone should be aware of, I believe. I share my story with you further on.

Again, I wish you the best of health – which you control!

Love, water and garlic,

Isabell VanMerlin
(I also changed my name.)
Dover, New Hampshire
Fall 2019

BODY SPEAK

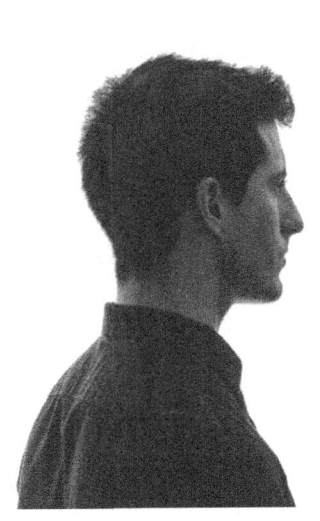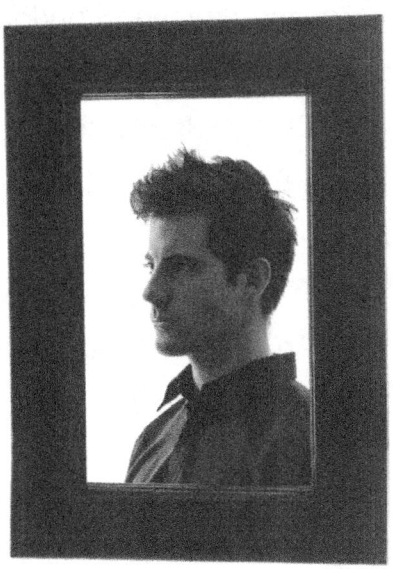

What do you really see when you look in the mirror?

INTRODUCTION

SPECIAL NOTE on DOWSING YOURSELF

This book was originally written as a guide for dowsing and tracking down the root causes of symptoms in *other* people. But what about your/my self? A friend JUST (on New Year's Day 2020) asked me, "How can I use this to dowse my own symptoms?"

Well, duh – you know what 'assuming' means …
I guess I thought you were smart enough to figure it out. But what it really means is that I wasn't smart enough to keep you from having to figure it out! Let me tell you now.

So, think of dowsing yourself as remote viewing or remote dowsing someone else. See yourself in your mind's eye, as you would see another person if you were doing this over the phone, for example. Use your fingers or a dowsing tool and follow the same steps.

BE SURE TO GET PERMISSION FROM YOURSELF.

BE SURE YOU ARE CLEAR AND WILL NOT BE INFLUENCING YOUR OWN ANSWERS.

Then go for it! To your own best health!

BODY SPEAK

GAYATRI

*You, who are the source of all power,
whose rays illuminate the whole world,
illuminate also my heart
so that it too can do your work.*

from The Book of Runes
Commentary by Ralph Blum

CHAPTER ONE
THE BASICS

A. MUSCLE TESTING

The "tool" that I use to dowse the body with is my fingers: muscle resistance analysis or applied kinesiology. Of course you may use a pendulum, bobber, or even rods, if they are your tools of choice. The first edition of *Body Speak* was spiral bound so it would lie flat, when open, and you could use the charts and diagrams directly from the book, the person being in front of you or at a remote location. I trust you will be able to use a clear plastic book stand or create a setup that will allow you to use your hands while looking at the charts in this second edition.

If you are a brand-new dowser, I highly recommend that you read *Letter to Robin* by Walt Woods, or ask a dowser to teach you some dowsing techniques – and jump right in. *Letter to Robin* is available from the American Society of Dowsers bookstore; you can also download it for free from the internet.

BODY SPEAK

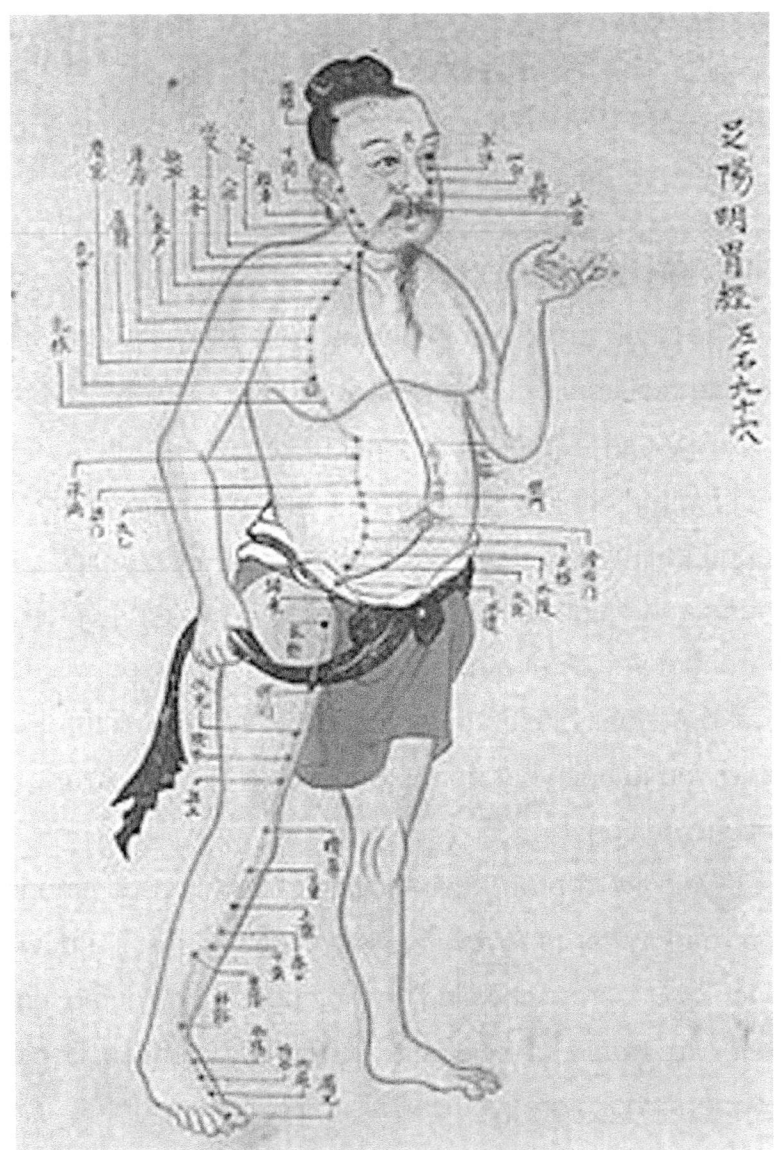

Chinese acupuncture points

THE BASICS

Muscle testing is not a new technique. Chiropractors have been using muscle testing for years to determine deficiencies in the body's nerve, muscle and skeletal structures. They usually use our arm- or leg-muscles, though, to see how strong our resistance is to a given question. I think fingers are easier, and less cumbersome to use.

We know that the brain sends electrical impulses to the various parts of the body to move muscles that move limbs, digest food and deliver nutrients to the proper places for the body's use, and to send hormones or enzymes to glands and organs in order for the body to function as an integrated, efficient unit.

Acupuncturists use very specific locations on the body, spots that have been pinpointed over millennia as reference points to glands and organs. The electricity from the brain flows to these points which are usually closely related to the physical location of the glands and organs. A healthy or normal acupuncture point is about the size of the head of a thumbtack. When an organ or gland is ill or diseased, however, the brain sends an enormous amount of electricity to that part of the body in order to heal or at least compensate

BODY SPEAK

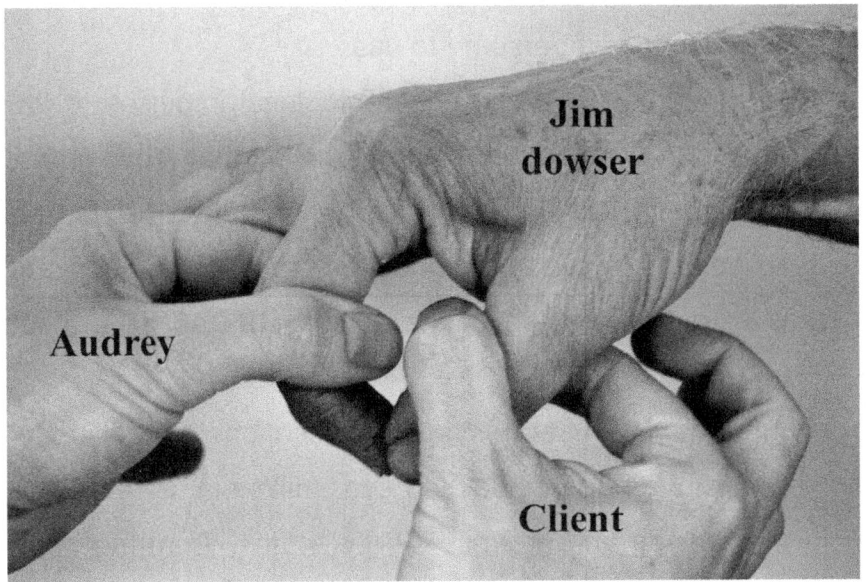

for its dysfunction. When that happens, the corresponding point becomes as large as a baseball, easily read as a "hot spot."

We will be using muscle testing at acupuncture points to find the "hot spots," just as an electrician would use an amp meter to measure an electrical circuit. It is an extremely simple and straightforward method – and efficient!

To begin, make a circle with the thumb and forefinger of your non-dominant hand, e.g., if you are left-handed, make a circle with the thumb and forefinger of your right hand. Your right hand will be the "positive terminal" or dial hand and your left hand will be the "negative terminal" or probe hand. If you are right-handed, then make the circle of your fingers with your left or dial hand, as the face or dial of the 'amp meter.' Jim and Audrey are dowser and client, respectively, in these next photos, so I will use their names instead of 'you' and 'the person.'

Jim is using his probe hand to touch the various acupuncture points of the body while Audrey, being tested, uses her fingers on the loop of his amp meter or dial hand to "test" the circuit.

BODY SPEAK

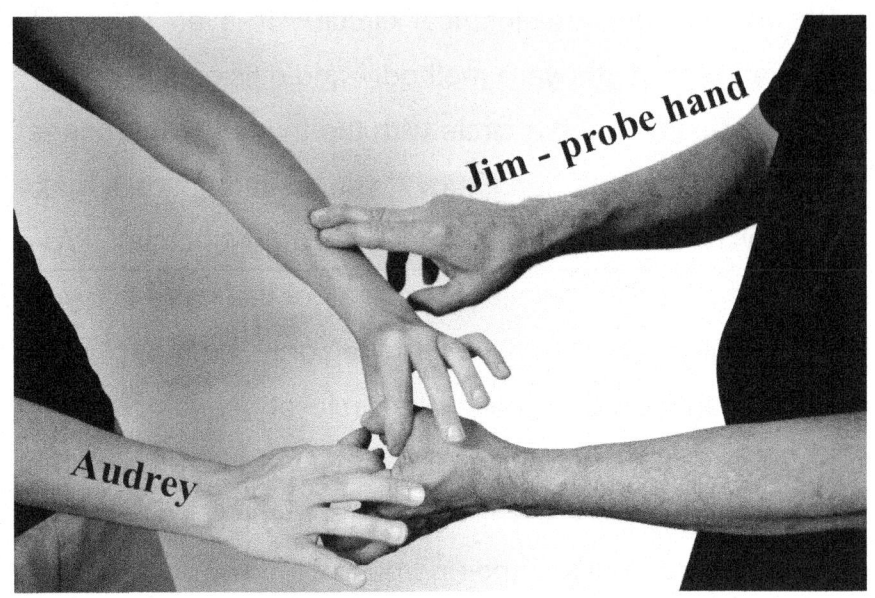

THE BASICS

So, Jim has his dial hand extended to Audrey and she has the forefingers and thumbs of both her hands making loops on his thumb and forefinger loop – all at the ready to test the point that Jim's probe hand is touching. An electrical circuit is completed when his probe hand touches Audrey and she pulls his finger loop. (When you are touching the spot and have that spot in your mind, you ask the person to "pull" with their fingers on your finger loop, thereby testing the resistance of your muscles for that particular spot.) If the finger loop remains strong and does not break apart with the pulling, that means that the point is strong and healthy; it is functioning properly. If, however, *your* fingers cannot resist the tension of the pulling of their fingers and the loop breaks open, then you have found a "hot spot," or a point that is receiving a great deal of electricity from the brain thus causing the spot to enlarge and wave its distress flag at you. YOUR finger muscles are relaying the message of how much or how little electricity is flowing to a particular point by how well they resist (or do not resist) their pulling on them.

BODY SPEAK

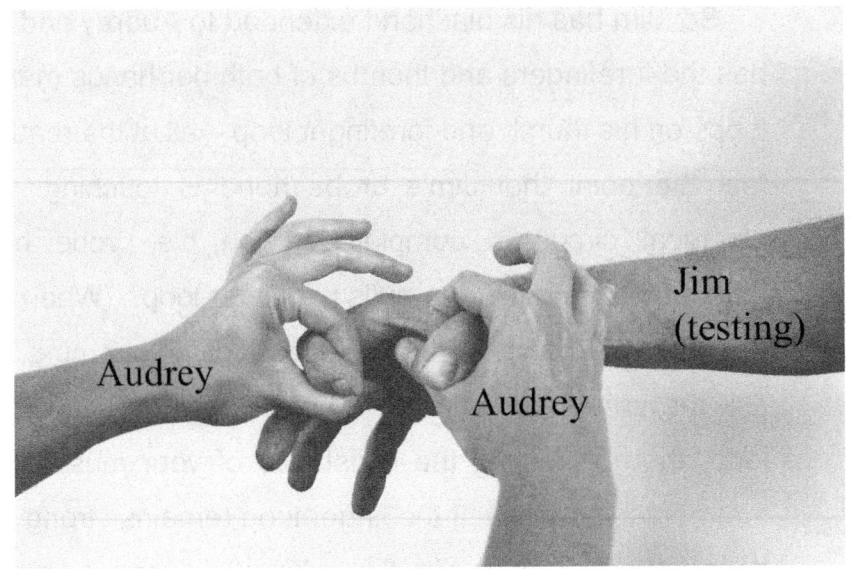

Found a hot spot!

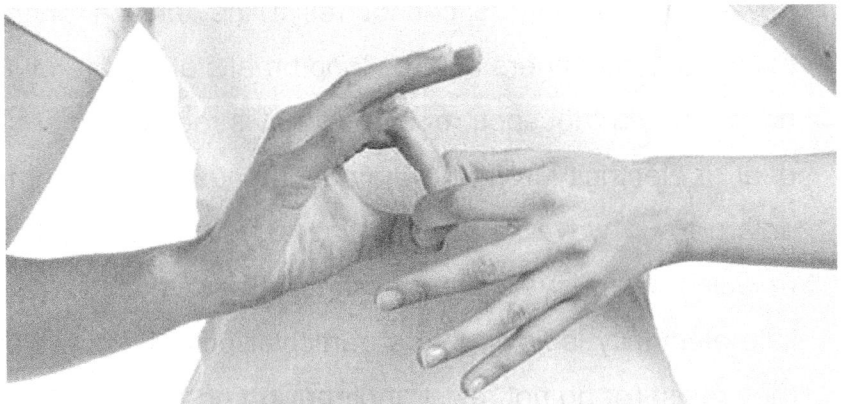

For self testing: use two finger loops or two fingers inside a loop
(or any other variation that works for you!)

THE BASICS

You may have to practice a little with the person you are testing so that they can get the feel of the proper amount of tension to apply to your finger loop: enough to make a valid test, but not so much as to rip your fingers off! A nice, firm pull, lasting approximately one-half second, will work well.

If you wish to test a person by remote viewing and still use your fingers, let your probe hand be the testing hand and insert the forefinger and middle finger of the probe hand inside the loop created by the thumb and forefinger of your dial hand. Instead of having the person "pull," open the fingers of your probe hand while you visualize the acupuncture point in your mind and ask if it is strong. It works the same way. If the point is strong and healthy, your dial-hand finger loop will stay strong. If the point or gland is being bombarded with electricity, your fingers will fly apart demonstrating the weakness of that point.

You can also use a pendulum or other tool for remote viewing using one hand to touch the point on the chart or diagram on the left pages in this book and the other hand to hold the dowsing tool.

BODY SPEAK

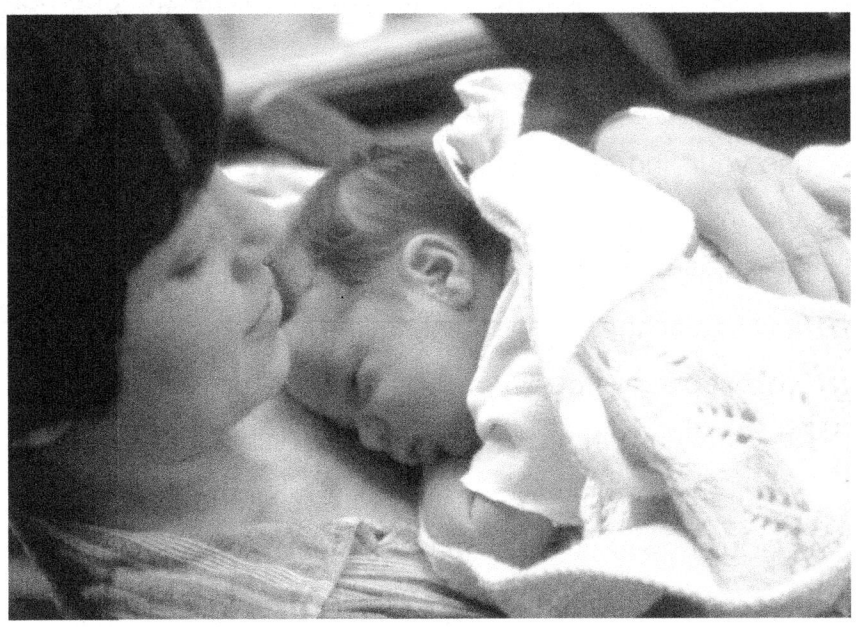

Four days old

B. INTENTION: Root Cause

A warning: the psyche can, and will, play tricks on you; the psyche is literal and will not read nuances or subtleties into your questions that seem obvious to you! My favorite story of psyche-play is the one of when I was pregnant with my daughter.

Sia's due date was June 3. Two weeks after June 3rd, I was getting bigger and bigger, and more and more awkward, and more and more impatient for my pumpkin to be born. Well, Dr. King hypnotized me and said, "Starting tomorrow, Thursday, as Day One, count how many days until Sia is born." I duly counted five days: Thursday, Friday, Saturday, Sunday, Monday, which meant she would be born on Monday. Well, I'm not sure what my psyche objected to about giving me the correct date, but she was NOT born five days after that particular night I started counting from, but rather a WEEK and FIVE DAYS later, or MONDAY, June 27, 1977!

BODY SPEAK

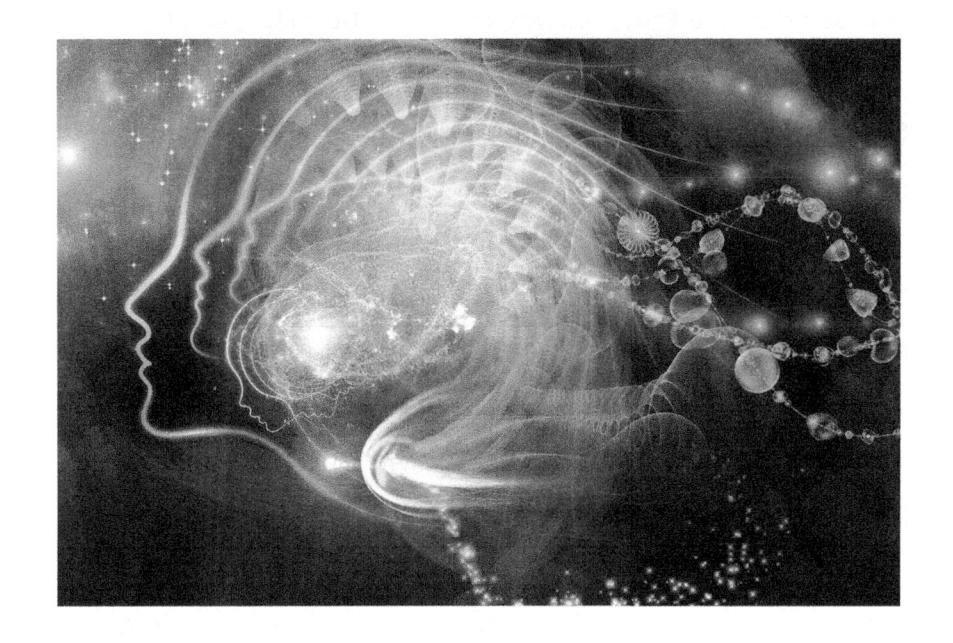

THE BASICS

Was Dr. King not precise enough in the way he asked the question? Did my psyche not want me to know the exact date for some reason? Was I being protected – or was my daughter being protected? If I had known that it was going to be almost two more weeks before she was born, would I have done something rash and possibly detrimental to our health? I don't know, but I do trust the process and my own dowsing ability enough now that I do not question the outcome as much as I used to when an answer is unexpected or appears to be "wrong." I usually get an answer, sooner or later, that demonstrates the "accuracy" of the answers I receive. I trust much more that Spirit, or the Universe, or God, always gives me the best – if I ask for it – answer, and expect it.

BODY SPEAK

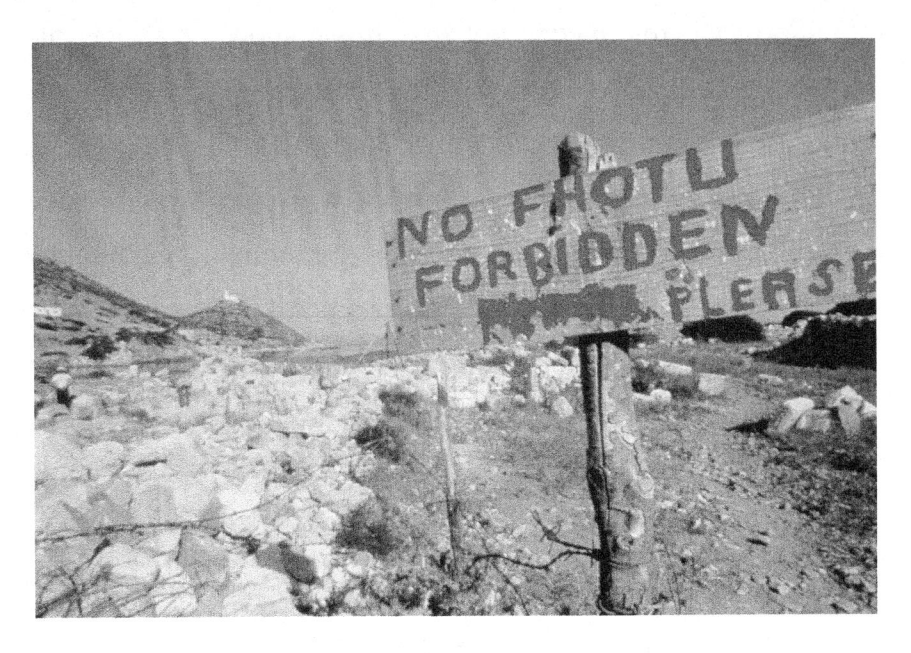

Ask permission before "trespassing"!

C. PERMISSION?

There are several perspectives on asking permission before dowsing . . . anything. Some dowsers feel it is unnecessary to ask permission because their intent is the highest good for all concerned. However, it might not be the best thing for the particular individual. The "traditional" questions of "Can I?" "May I?" and "Should I?" are certainly pertinent here, in my opinion. And I have added another question that I believe is even more important: "Does this person want to heal?"

I was very naïve when I started working as a holistic health practitioner. I guess I thought that if a person came to me and asked me to find the cause of their problem, then they really wanted to find out what the problem was and, therefore, wanted to fix it. I was wrong. I now believe that most people seeking help want someone else to fix them. It is very frustrating for a person like me to have answers to questions and solutions to problems and then discover the very people who have asked the questions or posed the problems are not interested in the solutions because they would have to be responsible for themselves *and* be open to receive healing. I can only show them a way to do that.

BODY SPEAK

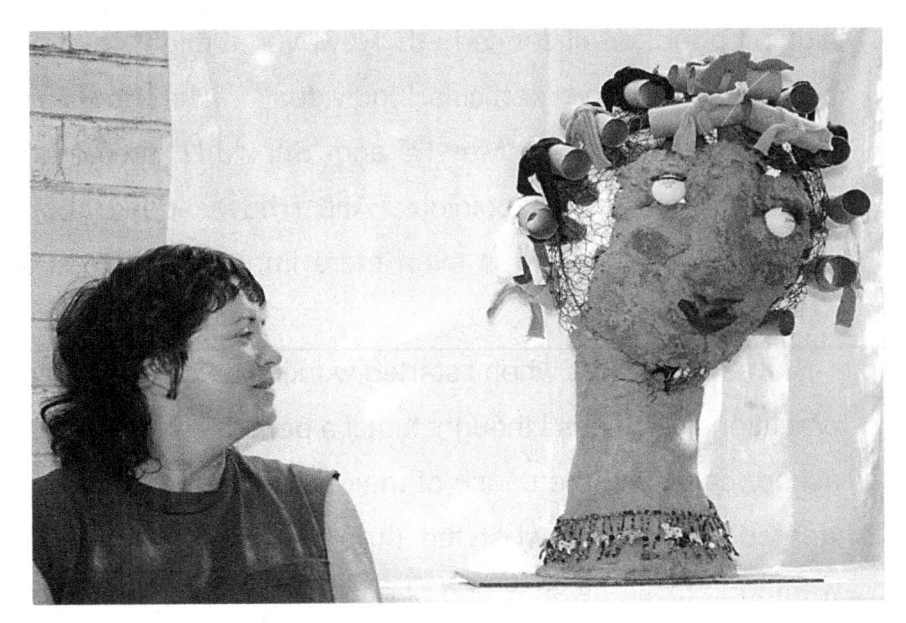

We are NOT empty-headed.

THE BASICS

My teacher, Sarah Meredith, had a questionnaire that she gave all her new clients. It had the statement "I am willing to take responsibility for my health," with four possible responses to choose from:

- a.   I am totally responsible for my health.
- b.   I am partly responsible for my health.
- c.   My health is a result of my environment.
- d.   I have no control over my health.

I quickly learned about the whiners/victims who, on the surface, came to me with genuine health problems, with the genuine desire to get better, if not completely well. But when they answered the question with anything less than "a," it became apparent that there was greater benefit to them in having a health problem than being in good health.[2] And my very own, self-same mother, who so eagerly healed herself of an ovarian tumor when she was in her mid-30s, died of the exact same malignancy 40 years later. It was only when I visited her on her death bed that I realized she had grown weary of this life and of the earthsuit she was wearing and had relinquished her desire to live. It was one of those great moments of clarity for me.

---

[2] Caroline Myss: *Why People Don't Heal and How They Can.*

BODY SPEAK

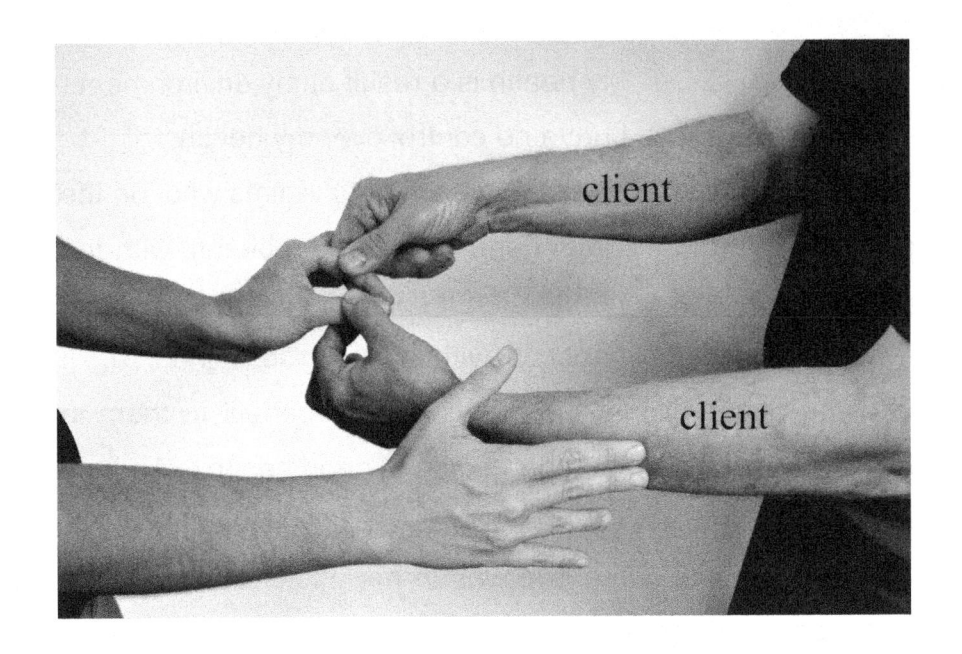

THE BASICS

By asking permission to dowse, and receiving a positive response, not only do you clear the way, but you are much more likely to get the "correct" answers. There is an infinite number of variations on this theme. For example, you may get permission to dowse only to discover, after all your work, that the person is going to do nothing with the information – or even more frustrating, do the exact opposite of the suggestions you might give! I try to keep in mind that we are all here to heal, but today might not be the day the person I am working with wants to heal. Or, that the healing might be MY healing and not my client's. Sigh. The mirror is everywhere, . . . is everyone.

I place my probe hand on the person's forearm; that is the permission "point" for me. And I have the permission questions "programmed" into my consciousness so that when I touch the person's arm, I make it the first "point" to test and I am asking permission in the form of "Can I?" "May I?" "Should I?" and also asking if they want to heal. If I get a negative response, I ask the questions individually in order

BODY SPEAK

KEEP
YOUR
OPINION
OUT
OF
IT !

THE BASICS

to get more information so that I can tell the person something of why I am not able to test them. Sometimes a negative response is merely a matter of the person not being hydrated. A drink of water will fix that right up. Another possibility is that the person may not be mentally or energetically present at the moment and a little reminder of what you are attempting to accomplish will bring the person back into their physical body and you may proceed with the testing.

Or, you may not get permission to test and you will have to let it go! It will be up to you, in that situation, to ask the person what's going on, or . . . . . fill in the blank! It will almost certainly be fear of some kind, but it could be deeply buried. Letting go might be the perfect solution to opening *your* mind and heart for the perfect answer.

BODY SPEAK

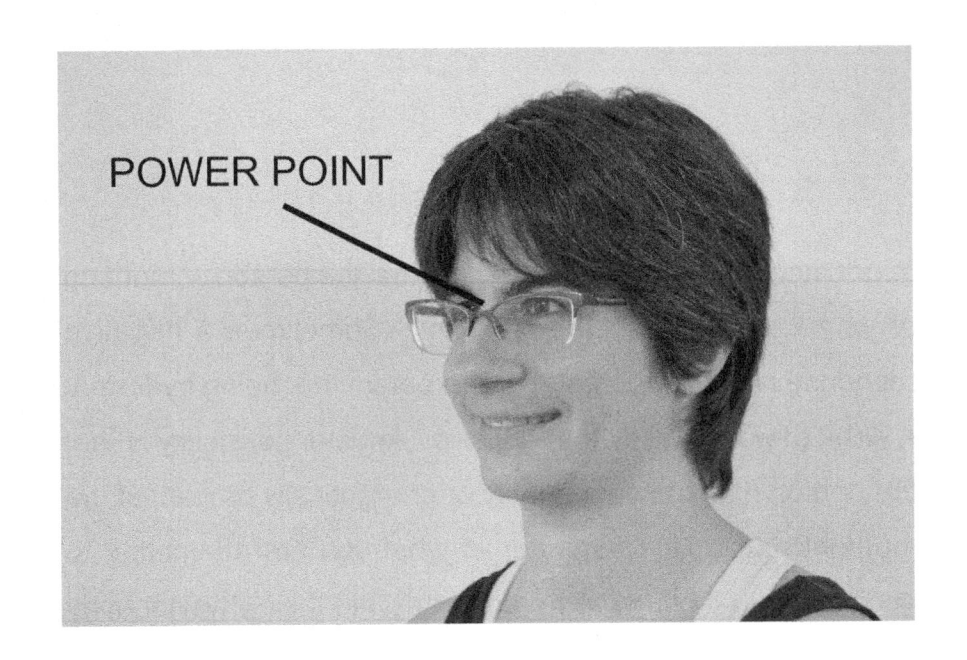

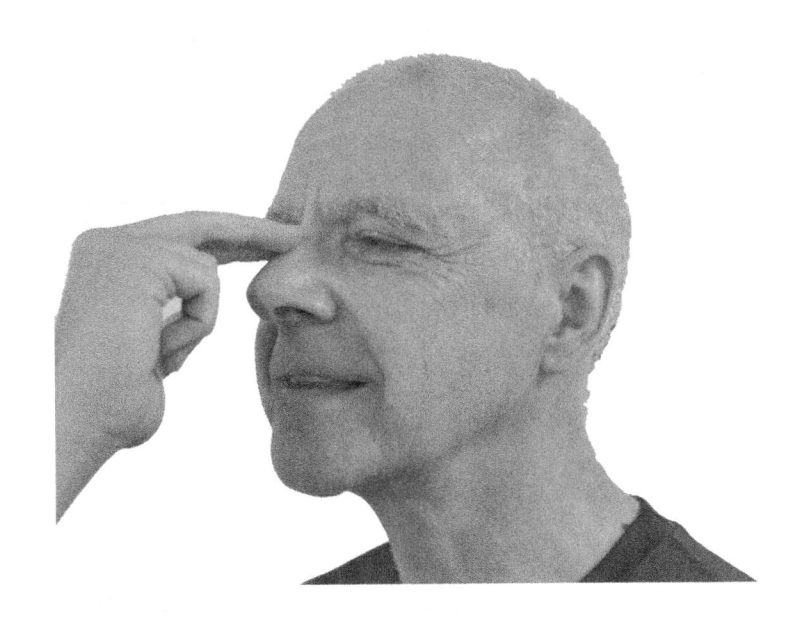

POWER POINT

D. POWER ON?

The second point to test is the "power" button at the very top of the nose. Use two fingers of your probe hand – forefinger and middle finger, or middle and ring fingers, close together – so that you have both positive and negative poles represented. Look at the photo on the opposite page: when you use two fingers in this way you are getting both energies: positive and negative. The polarized nature of our bodies and their atoms play an integral part of the testing. Sometimes we will use two fingertips together, representing the positive and negative, other times we will test for the positive and negative separately by using the palm of the hand for the positive, then the back of the hand for the negative. A memory trick: the Palm of the hand is Positive and the back of the hand, or the kNuckle or the Nail side of the hand is Negative.

When you touch the bridge of the nose with your fingers and ask the person to "pull," if his "power" is on, or his electromagnetic circuitry is functioning in a manner that makes him testable, your fingers will fly apart. This is the one point that appears to give you a negative response when, in fact, it is telling you that you can proceed. The reason is that this point is the power center of the body's whole electrical

BODY SPEAK

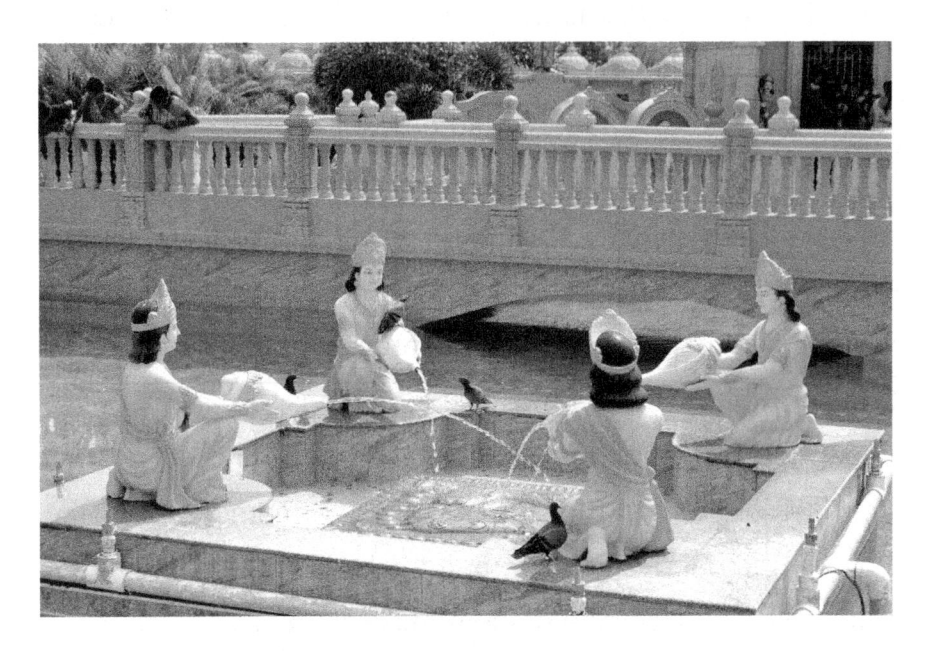

Nilkanthdham Swaminarayan Temple
on the banks of the Narmada River
Gujarat, India

THE BASICS

system. From this spot emanates any surplus electricity needed for healing or repairing, so its inherent power will make your fingers "blow."

If this spot does NOT blow, there are a couple of remedies I know of to turn power on again: 1) use your same probe fingers and flip your hand over and back: palm side up, then back side up; palm side up, then back side up several times, then test again. Often, that will "prime" the pump, and the power will come on again. 2) Another thing that can shut the power off is dehydration. Give the person a glass of water – and make sure YOU have enough water in your system also – to make the circuits operable. Water, the main ingredient in our bodies, is a great electrical conductor. Without enough water, lots of things do not function properly in our bodies. I think I will say that again, in capital letters, even though this is not the solution chapter of the book: WITHOUT ENOUGH WATER, LOTS OF THINGS DO NOT FUNCTION PROPERLY IN OUR BODIES!!!!![3]

---

[3] Dr. Julian Whitaker, in the May 1995 issue of his newsletter "Health and Healing," says that 50% of ALL ALLERGIES could be CURED if people drank enough water! [emphasis mine]

BODY SPEAK

A Buddhist Zen master came to the United States on a tour. His guide took him to Coney Island. At lunchtime the Zen Master ordered a hot dog from a street vendor and paid with a $20 bill. The vendor took the $20 and shut it in his drawer.

Surprised, the Zen master asked where his change was. The vendor looked at him soberly and said,

"Change must come from within."

THE BASICS

Something that I particularly have to guard against in myself and my testing is that of prejudice, or "prejudging" the condition. Because I have some little scraps of information about health and illness and nutrition, I have to guard against thinking I know what the root cause is before I ever start testing. If someone comes to me complaining of indigestion and he shows up with a hamburger, French fries and a milkshake in his hands, it can be very difficult for me not to want to say, "Change your diet and then see if you have indigestion!" And/or, "Don't waste my time." I try to completely clear my mind when I start testing – and ask Spirit to help me receive the information I seek. When I clear my mind and am open to new ideas, I am usually amazed by the interesting and unexpected answers I receive.

You might be surprised to know that good humor can also throw you off the track. Levity and laughter cure ills. If you are having too much fun, telling jokes and laughing with the person you are testing – or if they are laughing at something – you may not find a root cause for anything because there IS NO PROBLEM at that time. You don't

Open Your Mind to Receive

by Catherine Ponder,
Unity minister and prosperity teacher

want your client to be in the slough of despond; but a pink cloud will not allow the cause of the symptom to be read. Other things are painkillers, aspirin, mood-altering drugs, and alcohol. You cannot expect to get an accurate reading when the body is "not itself." So you can always ask if the person you are testing is taking any medication. If the person IS or HAS taken medication within a few hours of your testing, ask the body if it can give you accurate results by ignoring the effects of the drug. If so, proceed as usual. If not, ask when you could test and get accurate results, e.g. "Can I test later today and get accurate results?" And refine the time as much as you need to.

    Once you know the power is on and permission is granted, you are on your way to discovery and recovery. Open your mind to receive the answers the body has to tell you. It will definitely speak – if spoken to!

BODY SPEAK

BASIC MUSCLE-TESTING POINTS

May I, Can I, Should I? Want to heal?	Blood Pressure
Polarity/On-Off	Lymph
Structural/Skeletal	Thymus
Stress	Heart
Heavy Metal	Lungs
Master Brain	Metabolic
Emotional	Liver
Hypothalamus	Gall Bladder
Pituitary-Anterior/Posterior	Stomach
Pineal	Hiatal Hernia
Thyroid: 1, 4, 3	Spleen
Adrenals	Kidneys
(system) Poison	Pancreas
Primary Disease Organisms	Intestines
Virus	Bone
Spiritual	Calcium=Lack or Buildup-4 points
Eyes	Ovaries
Ears	Fallopian Tubes
Sinus	Testicles
Hormones	Prostate
Allergies	Urethra
Blood	Breasts

Use this chart to write down the locations of the points and/or use it as a checklist.

THE BASICS

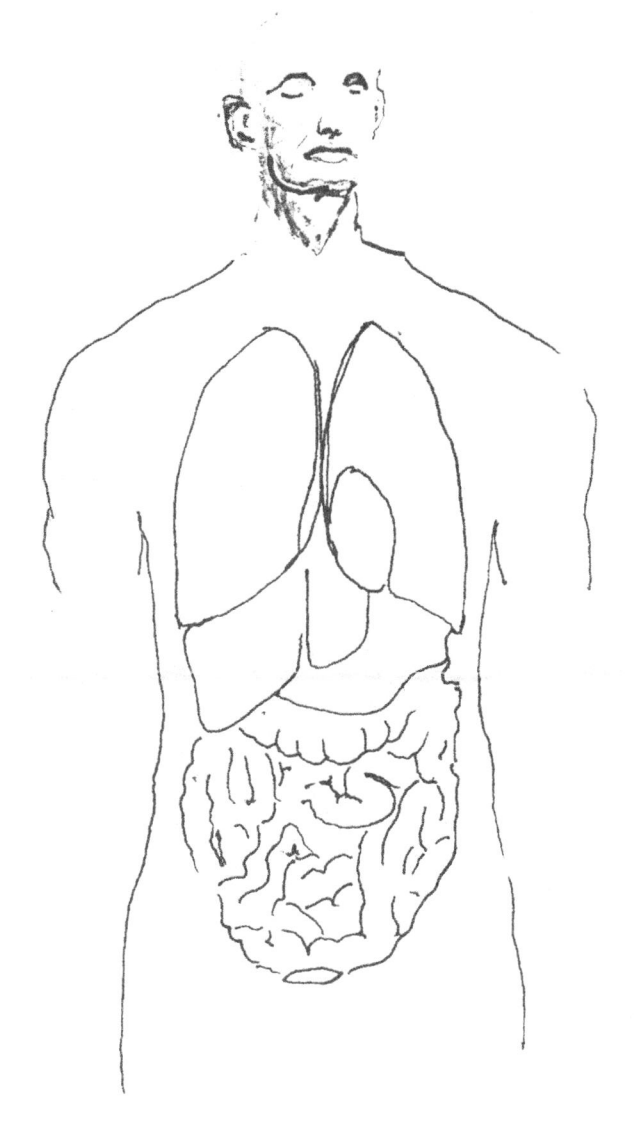

You can use this chart – or a copy of it – to mark the "hot spots."

BODY SPEAK

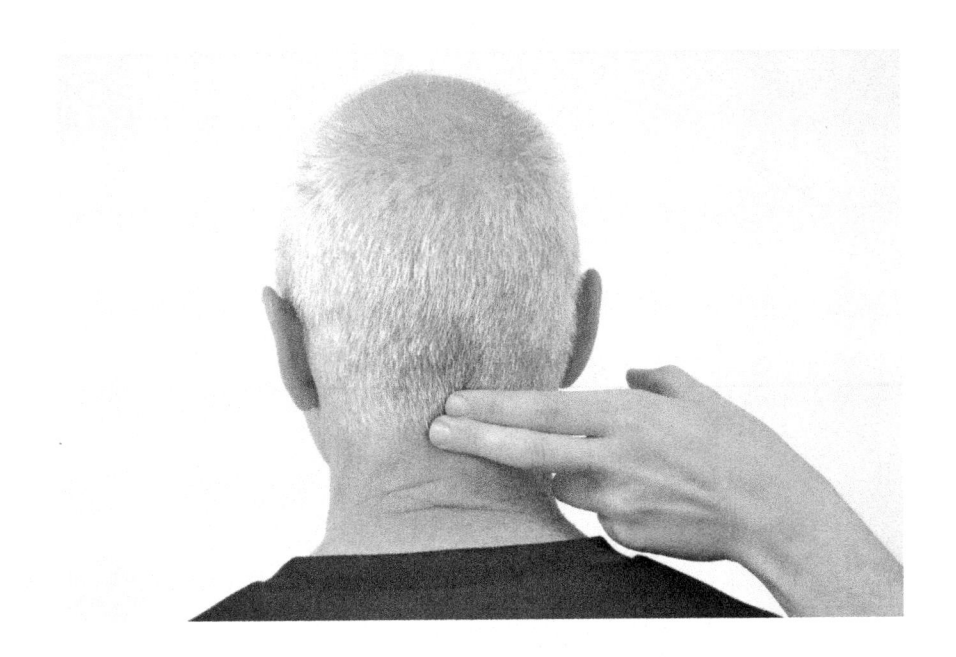

Structural/skeletal testing point

CHAPTER TWO
PRIMARY PHYSICAL POINTS

After you have focused on the intention of finding the root cause of the symptom, asked permission and having received a go-ahead, then checked the "power-on," you are ready to begin the testing of the actual points. We first look at the primary physical points. Quite often we will find the root cause among them. And quite often there is a chain of glands and organs, like a sequence of dominoes, that are affected by the root problem. We are only physically or consciously aware of the last "domino to fall," thereby causing the symptom. In actuality there are usually at least two, and as many as five, "dominoes" or malfunctions in between the root problem and its current manifestation or symptom.

After verifying that the power is on, the first point I always test is:

STRUCTURAL – Skeletal

This point is in the middle of the back of the neck. Place two fingers of the probe hand on the back of the neck, and ask the person to pull your fingers. If your fingers

Benne Seed Wafers
(Sesame Seed Cookies)

¾ c. sesame seeds
¾ c. butter
½ c. brown sugar
½ c. white sugar
1-1/4 c. whole wheat pastry flour
    (or whatever kind you happen to have)
    OR a gluten-free cookie mix
1 rounded tsp. baking powder
1 egg
1+ tsp. vanilla

Toast sesame seeds in a glass or heavy-bottomed saucepan or skillet. Add butter and let melt, then add sugar. Remove from heat and add flour, then the remaining ingredients. Drop by spoonful on cookie sheet. Bake 8 minutes at 325° F. (Baking time might vary if you are using a gluten-free mix.) Easy and nummy! This is a very forgiving recipe. If you want them more cakey, add more flour and egg; for thinner and crisper, use less flour – and only egg white? – more butter!

If you are making gluten-free cookies, follow the recipe on the box or flour mix and just add the toasted sesame seeds.

The rationale for these cookies is that sesame seeds contain lots of **calcium**!

break apart, it means that there is spinal or skeletal damage – from an accident or possibly from congenital defects (sometimes caused by drug abuse in one or both parents, e.g., thalidomide babies, years ago; opioids nowadays).

If the structural point blows, I usually suggest that the person seek out a chiropractor, after testing for the propriety of chiropractic help. If there has been an accident and the spine has been knocked out of alignment causing pinched nerves, a chiropractor's adjustments can be the perfect solution. And that usually is the end of a search when the structural point goes. Of course, I love to find out what the accident was – or how the genetic defect came to be! I'm nothing if not curious, and following my curiosity leads me down the path of experience, knowledge – and hopefully wisdom. Let your curiosity have its head and see where it takes you.

There is another thing you can ask when you find a person with skeletal or structural problems: "Is there any nutrition that would help this person?" By far the greatest problem among European-heritage people I have found in my practice is POOR ASSIMILATION of CALCIUM. Usually, we Americans get enough calcium in our diets that we do not

BODY SPEAK

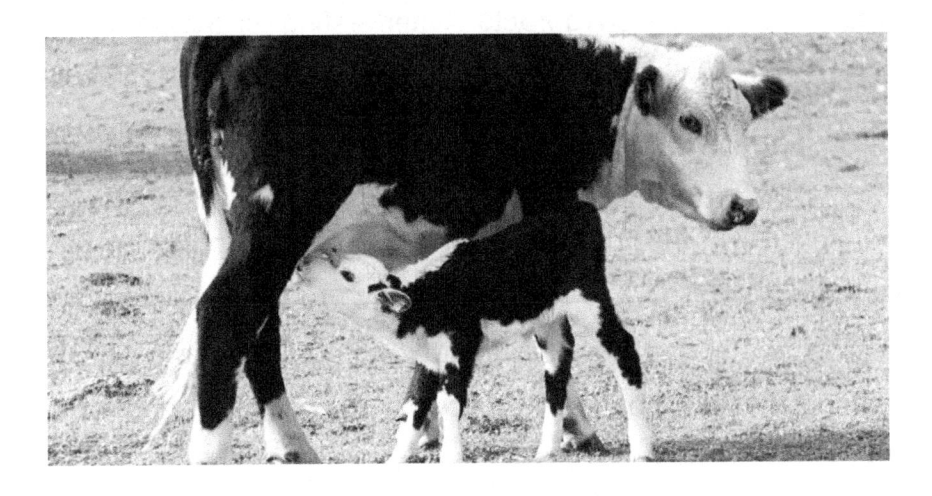

Cow's milk is for calves.
It is not designed for humans and
it's not a good source of calcium for us!

need to take supplemental calcium; the problem is that we do not assimilate the calcium we ingest – from whatever source. For people who have structural problems such as the spinal column pinching nerves causing pain or dysfunction, they might be relieved with chiropractic adjustment, but if they do not have enough calcium to maintain healthy synapses between nerves, and, thus, for the muscles to hold the adjustment in place, then the person's spine will very quickly slip back into its incorrect position and the same symptoms will manifest.

At this point in your examination I would ask if the person needs any nutritional support to maintain perfect health, and if the answer is yes, I would ask if calcium is needed. If so, see farther on in this chapter, pages 67 and 69, about the parathyroid and its role in the assimilation of calcium in the body. The probability of the parathyroid needing stimulation or supplementation is great.

BODY SPEAK

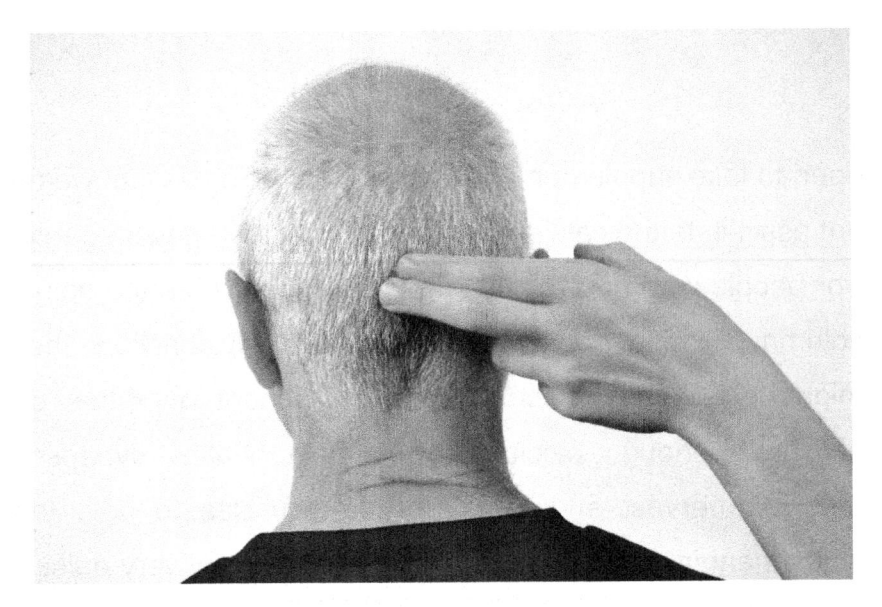

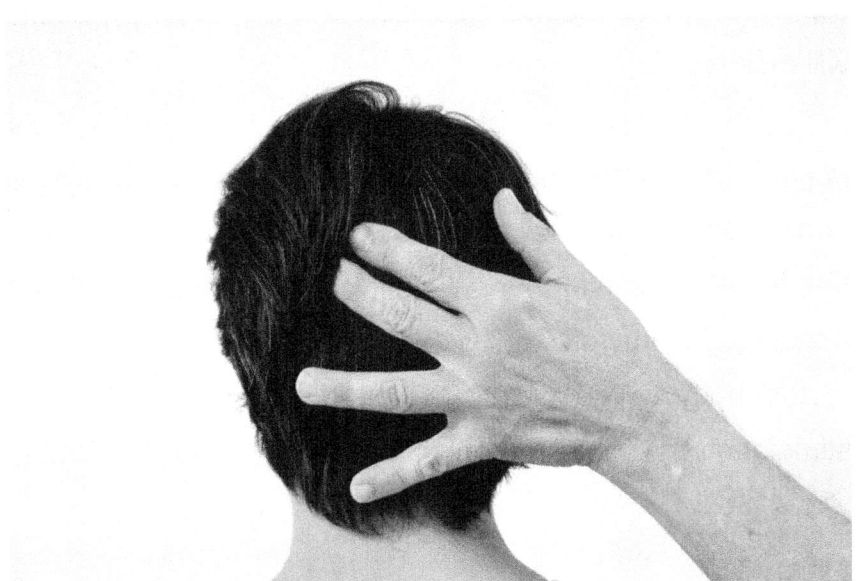

Stress testing point – just *above* occipital bump

PRIMARY PHYSICAL POINTS

STRESS

I was surprised that stress does not show up more often than it does, in *my* testing anyway, as a primary source of illness. And it rarely is a secondary or intermediary point. I believe, however, that "stress," as I think of it, shows up more often as an emotional body or spiritual body problem. Chapters 5 and 6 deal with those kinds of stress.

A good example of stress might be an auto mechanic who has to contort his body all day long to reach hard-to-get-to places in or under or around a car. Repeating a certain task for long periods of time can easily cause stress. Carpal tunnel syndrome might be caused by stress.

The point for testing stress is the back of the head, just above the occipital lump or bump or hump (the protuberance that caps the spinal column as it disappears into the skull).

When the prime (or root cause) point blows, I consciously acknowledge that fact and write it down, particularly if I wish to show the path to the person, or keep records on a client. (See diagram on next page.)

Root Cause

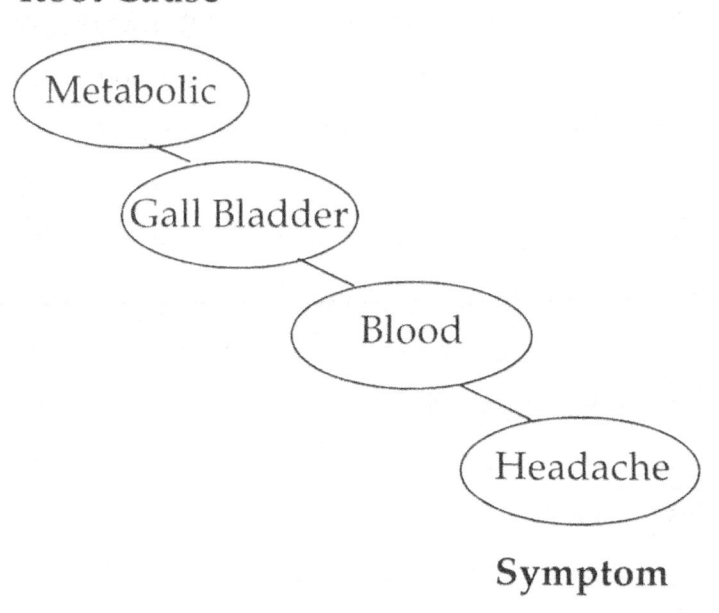

(Metabolic)
(Gall Bladder)
(Blood)
(Headache)

Symptom

PRIMARY PHYSICAL POINTS

I then rub the stress (or prime) point down using the same probe fingers and by giving two strokes with my fingertips or the pads of my fingers. The reason for rubbing the point down is to shut off the hot spot for a short period of time in order to find the intermediate spots that form the chain from root cause to symptom. Turning off the hottest spot allows the next "hottest" spot to be found with testing.

To find out if the root cause is the only cause of the symptom, rub the stress spot down and then test the symptom *area* to see if the connection is direct. For example, with the headache, the stress point was the first point to blow, so we know that is the root cause. Rub the stress point down and then touch the forehead or the temple, or wherever the headache is manifesting, and ask the person to pull. If that spot blows, then you know that stress is the root *and* direct cause of the headache. If the headache point holds strong, then go on to the other points that follow here, and in Chapter 3, until another one of them blows. Rub *it* down, in turn, and again try testing the headache area. This is how we find the succession of affected glands and organs that have finally resulted in the headache.

BODY SPEAK

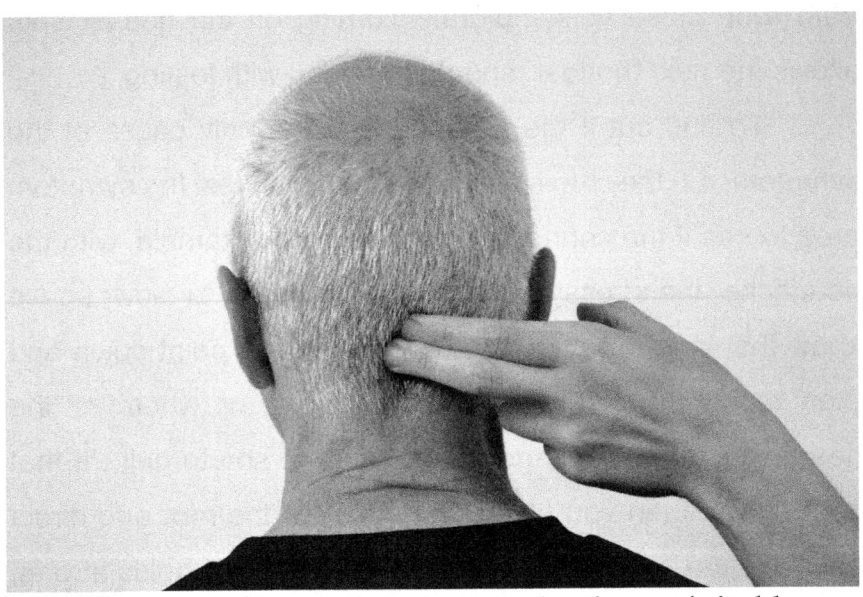

Heavy metal testing point – just *under* the occipital bump

Another example of stress might be when an (adult) child is taking care of an ailing parent. The stress is coming from an outside source – the aging parent - but it becomes a physical, mental and/or spiritual problem. The stressed person may not be getting enough sleep, which is a physical problem. There could be a brain imbalance, thus causing mental stress: "My father is quite old and cannot live forever. He will die, but I don't want him to." You can probably see in this example how "stress" could come from an emotional cause, made worse by poor nutrition (lack of calcium?) which puts stress on other organs, … etc.! When you get to the end of the chain, you might ask if some relief could be gained by using the Neuro Emotional Releasing Therapy in Chapter 6.

HEAVY METAL Toxicity

When this point blows it means the body has taken in too much heavy metal such as mercury or lead and is being poisoned by it. The source could be from a job: a welder, a jeweler, even a **dentist**, from handling such metals. I tested a man once whose heavy metal point blew and it turned out that he was a photographer and processed his own negatives

BODY SPEAK

Frequency of Symptoms
of mercury toxicity gained from analysis of questionnaires from 1,320 patients* pre-1988

73.3%	Unexplained irritability
72.0%	Constant or very frequent periods of depression
67.3%	Numbness and tingling in extremities
64.5%	Frequent urination during the night
63.1%	Unexplained chronic fatigue (today over 85%)
62.6%	Cold hands and feet, even in moderate/warm weather
60.6%	Bloated feeling after eating
58.0%	Difficulty remembering or use of memory
55.5%	Sudden, unexplained or unsolicited anger
54.6%	Constipation on a regular basis
54.2%	Difficulty in making even simple decisions
52.3%	Tremors or shakes of hands, feet, head, etc.
52.3%	Twitching of face and other muscles
49.1%	Experience frequent leg cramps
47.8%	Constant or frequent ringing or noise in ears
43.1%	Get out of breath easily
42.5%	Frequent or recurring heartburn
40.8%	Excessive itching
40.4%	Unexplained rashes, skin irritation
38.7%	Constant or frequent metallic taste in mouth
38.1%	Jumpy, Jittery, Nervous
37.3%	Constant death wish or suicidal intent (today over 90%)
36.4%	Frequent insomnia
35.6%	Unexplained chest pains
35.5%	Constant or frequent pains in joints
32.4%	Tachycardia
28.2%	Unexplained fluid retention
20.8%	Burning sensation on the tongue
20.1%	Get headaches just after eating
14.9%	Frequent diarrhea

*Data collected from the patients of Dr. Hal A. Huggins.
Recent increases may be related to 50X increase in Hg release from hi-Cu amalgam.

Compliments of Blanche Grube Enterprises D/B/A Huggins Applied Healing
Blanche D Grube, DMD, IMD Owner/President

and prints. His symptoms were general malaise, poor color (going from gray to bright pink, neither of which is a natural skin tone) and headaches. I urged him to detox with distilled, ionized water: a few drops UNDER the tongue, from a glass dropper or ceramic or wooden spoon, from a glass (not plastic) jar, every half-hour, if possible, for four days. If you have no other source of distilled water except a plastic grocery-store gallon jug, decant it into a glass jar and put it in the sun for a day or two – then it will be ionized. (Put the lid on very loosely, only to keep dust out.) Also, eating dark, leafy greens: spinach, kale, collard, turnip, mustard, dandelion, and romaine lettuce are VERY EFFECTIVE for combining with the metal and removing it from the body. Blue-green algae might also do the trick. Dowse for the effectiveness of the algae as it is very potent. I have never found the need for it in myself, but for my dog and other humans, definitely yes.

    Another source of heavy metal poisoning is amalgam fillings. Use all four fingertips and point to different parts of the jaws to test for secondary points. The chart on the opposite page lists symptoms from heavy metal poisoning in order of frequency of appearance.

BODY SPEAK

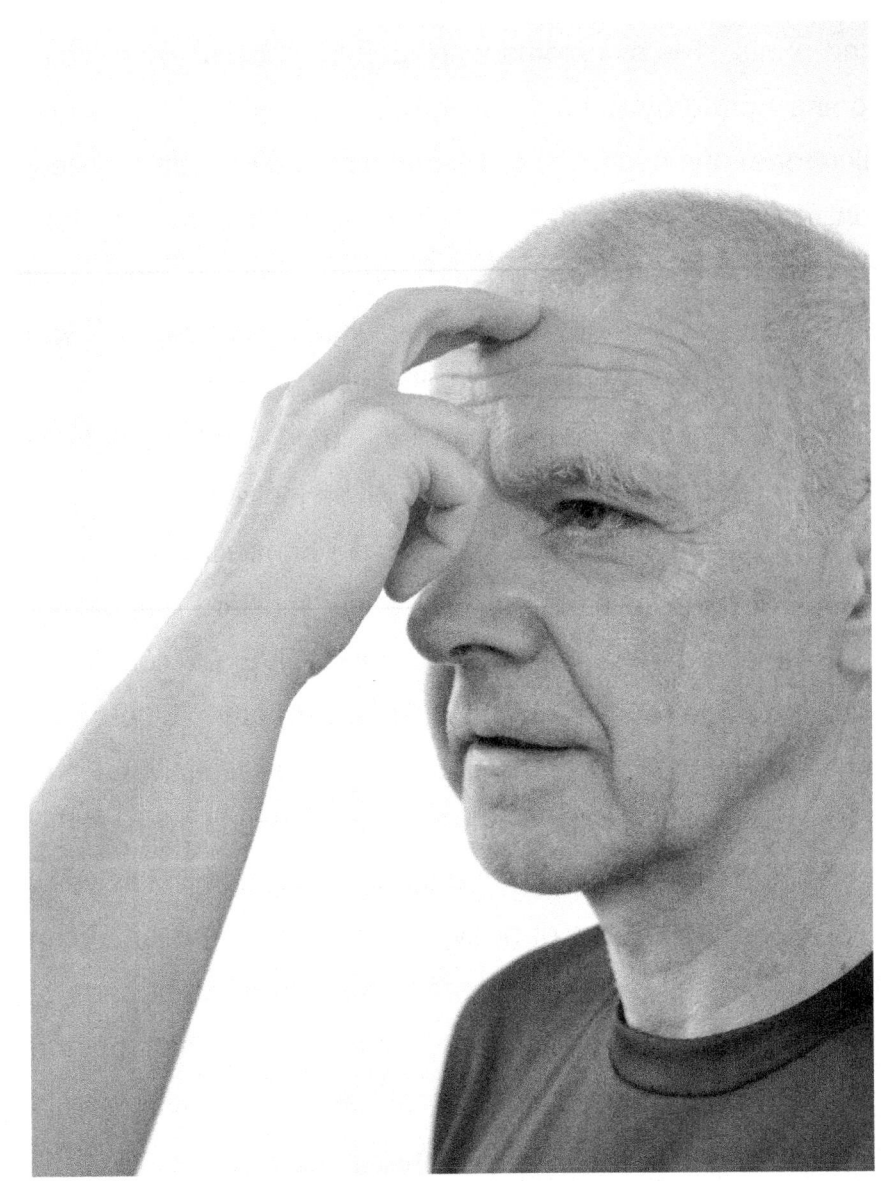

Master brain

PRIMARY PHYSICAL POINTS

The **MASTER BRAIN** point is at the hairline, in the middle: if you have a widow's peak hairline, the master brain point will be at the "peak." (Do I need to draw a map or make any disparaging remarks about people who don't still have hair at their hairline or what was their hairline?) (You may be surprised at the answers you receive if you dowse for the root cause of baldness in different people!) Master brain is the "headquarters" of the nervous system. The culmination of the spinal cord, the actual gray matter, is the point you are testing, but because it is the control center of the nervous system, the implications of illness of or trauma to some part of the brain are bound to be symptoms somewhere else in the body. If this point blows, rub the spot down **twice** and check the symptom point to see if the brain is the direct cause of the symptom. If the symptom point does not blow, then test other points for the intermediary points that are affected.

BODY SPEAK

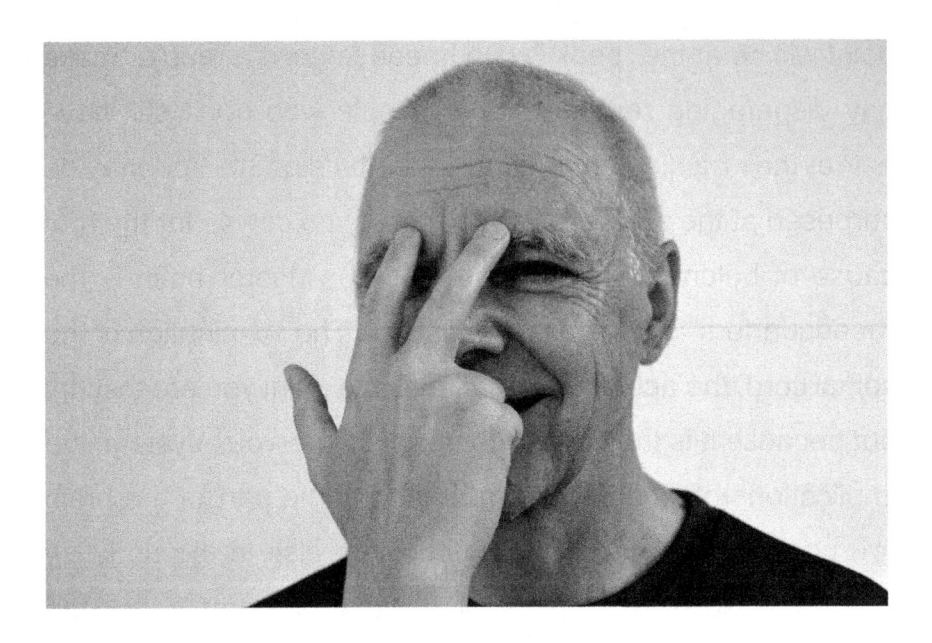

Emotional test point

PRIMARY PHYSICAL POINTS

EMOTIONAL test point. I put this point in here because the test location is between the master brain and hypothalamus points. This point is actually two points that you test at the same time, with two fingertips (I use my forefinger and middle finger.), separated into a V, at the brow, the beginning of the eyebrows, on either side of the third eye, as it were! See Chapter 4 if this point blows; it is different from the stress point and there is quite a lot one can do quickly and effectively for emotional dysfunction.

I don't usually test for intermediate points when the emotion point blows unless I am testing for more than one symptom. If you are testing for more than one symptom, test one at a time. However, when you find the root cause of one, you may ask if any other symptom is related to this one or its root cause. Sometimes seemingly unrelated symptoms come from the same dysfunction.

BODY SPEAK

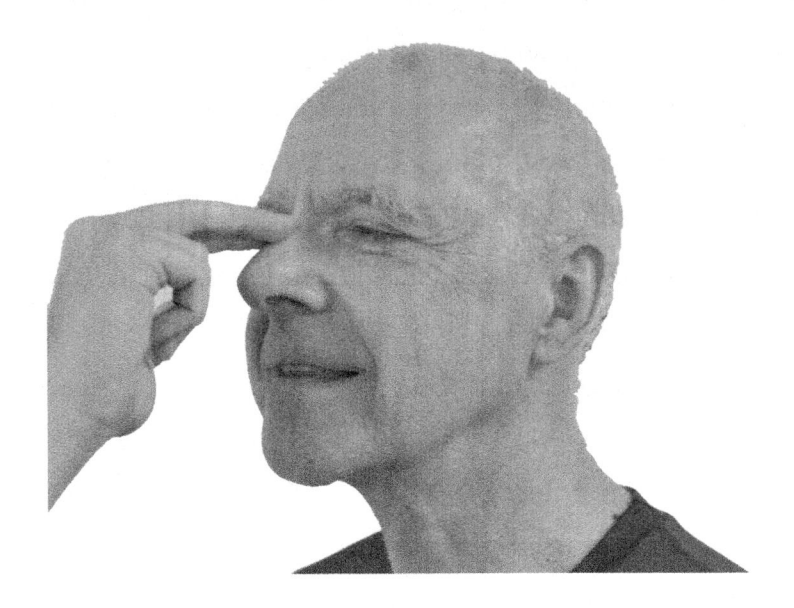

Hypothalamus

PRIMARY PHYSICAL POINTS

HYPOTHALAMUS: This point is a very important one and has turned out to be the location of many root causes in my experience. The middle of the nose, between the very tip of the nose and the bridge, or "power" point, is the testing location. Imagine a horizontal line going into the brain through the nose at that point, and another horizontal line going into the brain from the top of the ear, at a 90-degree angle to the nose line; the point at which they would intersect is where you will find the hypothalamus.

The hypothalamus is the master controller of the entire endocrine system. It regulates water in the cells, blood pressure, the heart, veins, kidneys, adrenals, pituitary, thyroid, parathyroid, lungs, liver, appetite, body temperature, sleep pattern, emotion, memory and concentration. All of our organs and glands receive hormones or enzymes or messages in some form from the hypothalamus, either directly or through an intermediate gland or organ. Symptoms of hypothalamus problems range from indigestion to diabetes, arthritis to heart disease, blindness to osteoporosis, uncontrolled heart rate to diverticulosis to unregulated body

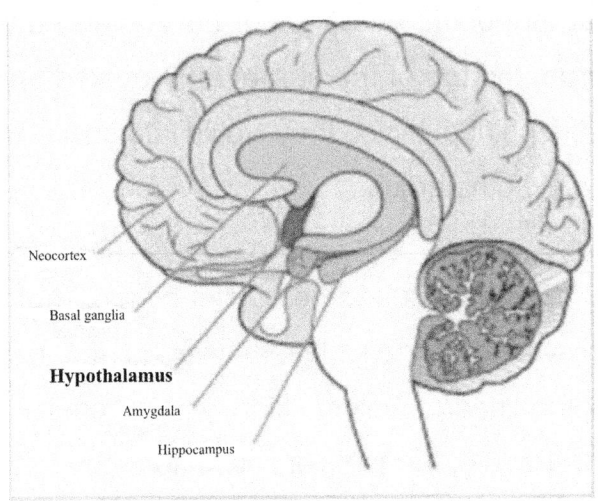

in the central-most part of the brain

temperature, bulimia, anorexia, and narcolepsy. I do not know of one medical doctor who tests the hypothalamus at all, even though they are very well aware of its extensive influence on the entire body. It is not an organ, but a part of the brain, and the fact that its location is so protected, i.e., the very center of the brain, farthest away from its outer protection, the skull or "brainbox," and is protected by the great bulk of our gray matter, are all excellent indicators of its importance to the body.

The testing of the hypothalamus is a little unusual in that you want the client to pull continuously for up to ten seconds. Tell this to the person before you start this point so he will not give a quick pull and release. Count out loud to ten, slowly, so that you will be giving each count a second. If the hypothalamus is going to blow, it may blow right away at one or two, which will mean that there is serious trauma to the hypothalamus or that it is an acute condition at this time. If your fingers do not release until eight or nine, then the condition is less severe, has not been in existence very long, or might be in the process of healing.

BODY SPEAK

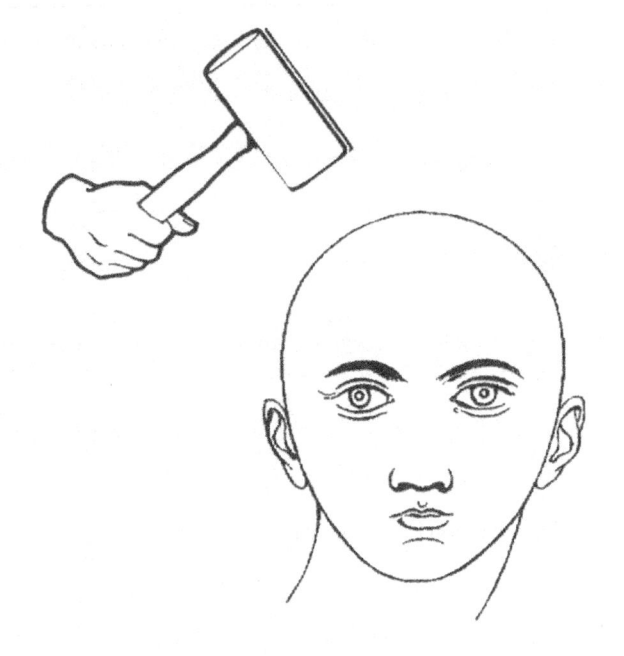

Who is holding the hammer? Or what does it represent?

PRIMARY PHYSICAL POINTS

I have many stories in my repertoire about the hypothalamus. One woman I tested confirmed that her hypothalamus condition was inherited before I could even ask her out loud. I had already received a positive response to the question – but she didn't know that I had asked her body! Another hypothalamus condition came from a very severe blow to the head in a young man who had not connected his symptoms to the head injury he received in an auto accident; the timing, however, was too coincidental to be discounted.

When I lived in Tucson and was doing a great deal of body dowsing, I found the water in Tucson, whose quality is dubious, at best, and is filled with chemicals, at worst, to be a major cause of hypothalamus dysfunction. Lesions are created on the hypothalamus. I do not know the physiology of this phenomenon, but I certainly would be interested in hearing from anyone who has more information.

BODY SPEAK

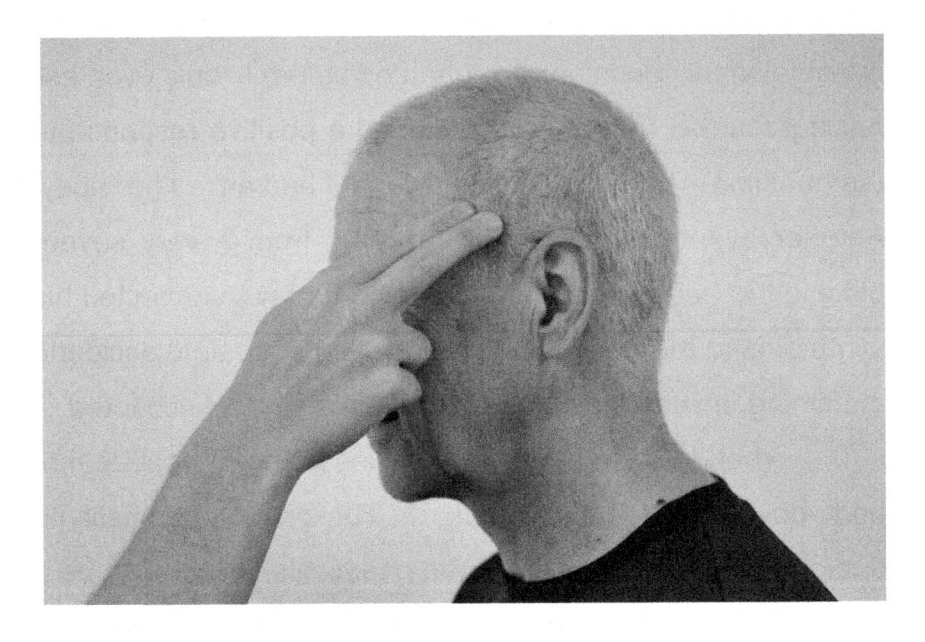

Pituitary gland – posterior point

PRIMARY PHYSICAL POINTS

PITUITARY GLAND: The pituitary regulates growth. It is controlled by the hypothalamus and controls the thyroid. It has two nodules: anterior and posterior, and the test sites are the temples, just beyond the eyes. It is in front of the hypothalamus and is a gland, not part of the brain. The anterior nodule is tested by touching the client's head with two fingertips on the left temple, and the posterior by touching the right temple.

BODY SPEAK

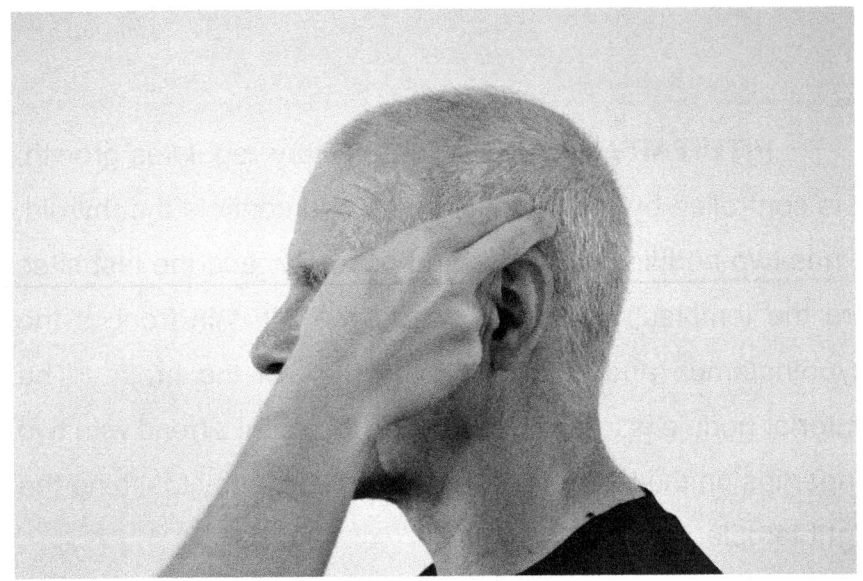

Pineal gland

PINEAL GLAND: The pineal gland is a neighbor of the hypothalamus and the pituitary nodes. Since I am right handed, my probe hand is my right hand, and I use a point on the left side of my client's head for testing. The spot is the side of the head – behind the spots for the pituitary points, directly over the top of the ears. If you are left-handed, use the same point on the right side of your client's head, as the gland is in the center of the skull and your intention is to test the pineal gland, thus you will be able to find the enlarged field from either side of the head if it is receiving extra amounts of electrical energy for some dysfunction.

The pineal gland is something of a mystery as far as its function in the human body. It has been thought of as the vestigial third eye, even the seat of the soul. It affects our spirituality. We do know that it has to do with the body's clock such as jet lag and hormonal imbalances, particularly in women and their menstrual cycles – at least those are manifestations of dysfunction of which I am aware. There are some birds whose pineal glands serve as a timing device.

Light: fluorescent light, natural light, moonlight, neon signs and radiation (from high-altitude flying) all seem to be

BODY SPEAK

Wealth
Purple
or Burgundy
Wood
Hipbone
Eldest Daughter

**Fame/Integrity/
Community Involvement**
Red
Fire
Eye
Middle Daughter
Summer

Marriage & Partnership
White & Red
or Pink
Earth
Internal Organs
Mother & Sister

Family & Friends/Ancestors
Green
Wood
Foot
Eldest Son
Spring

Center — Earth — Yellow — **Health**

Children/Creativity
White
Metal
Mouth
Youngest Daughter
Autumn

**Knowledge/
Self-Cultivation**
Dark or Midnight Blue
Earth
Knowledge
Hand
Youngest Son

Career
Black
Water
Ear
Middle Son
Winter

**Beneficial People/
Travel**
Grey or
Black & White
Metal
Head
Father & Brother

◁   △   ▷

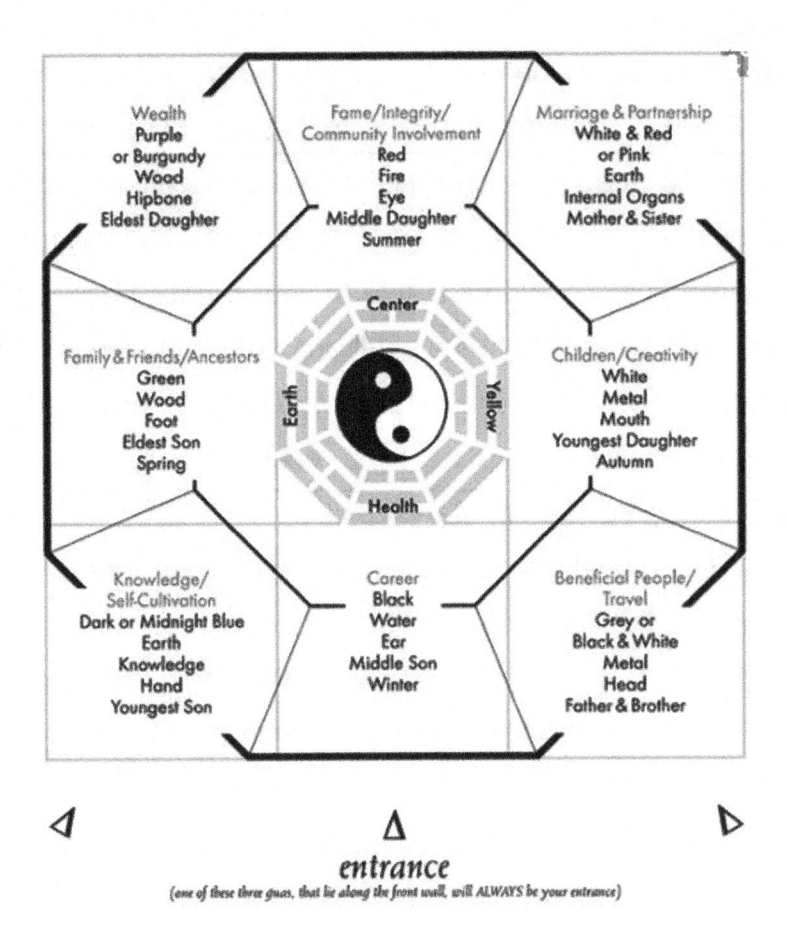

entrance
(one of these three guas, that lie along the front wall, will ALWAYS be your entrance)

The Bagua (or octagon) of Feng Shui is used to organize the energy of your living and/or working space.

PRIMARY PHYSICAL POINTS

be major influences on the pineal gland despite its location inside the skull and under the gray matter of the cerebrum.[4] A very interesting book having to do with women, the moon and their (respective and "symbiotic") cycles is *Lunaception* by Louise Lacey. I am not aware of any particular nutrition that helps the pineal gland other than that of glandular extracts and of generally building the immune system, except that my brother, an airline pilot, found that taking garlic capsules relieved him of jet lag!

If the pineal gland turns out to be the prime point in a testing, by all means ask all the questions you can think of to see if nutrition and/or light/colored light therapy will help. You might want to ask if Feng Shui (the Chinese Sacred Art of Placement) would help discover noxious zones in the person's home or office, or if there are street lights or neon signs that are disturbing the pineal gland – or even lots of air travel with its subsequent radiation from being in a thinner atmosphere – that might be stressing this important gland. There are some good books out on this subject now.

---

[4] *The Ancient Art of Color Therapy* by Linda Clark has an intriguing chapter on sitting under colored lights to heal certain problems; the object is definitely to "expose" the pineal gland to the lights.

BODY SPEAK

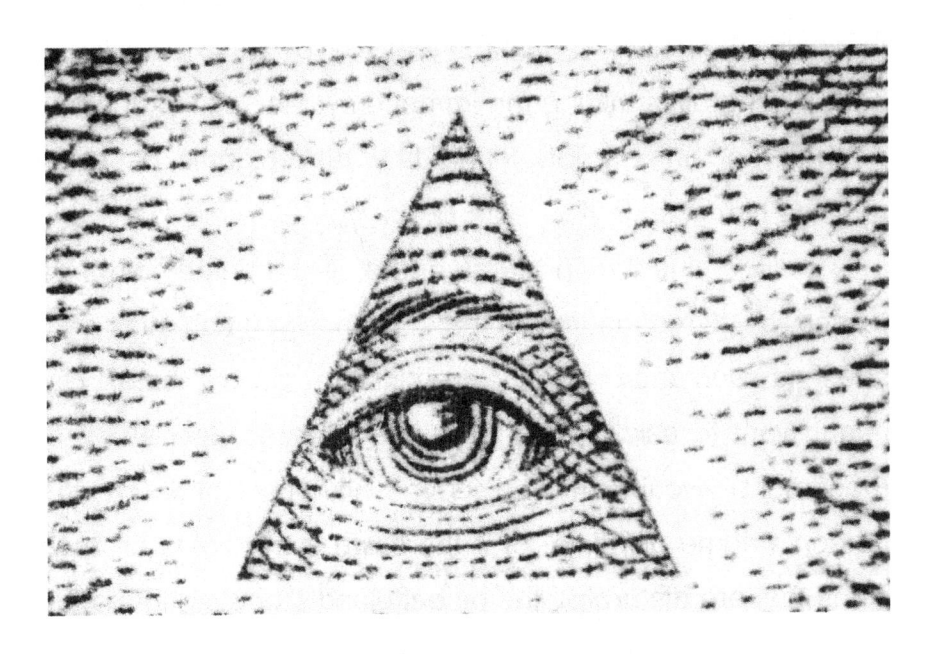

The all-seeing / third eye

PRIMARY PHYSICAL POINTS

Again, I find that I get excited thinking about the infinite number of possibilities of causes and cures, especially when it has been my experience that I am constantly confronted with unexpected information and answers. The general population of this planet provides us with an infinite variety of symptoms and causes to examine which means, to me, a lifetime of discovery. Wheee!

BODY SPEAK

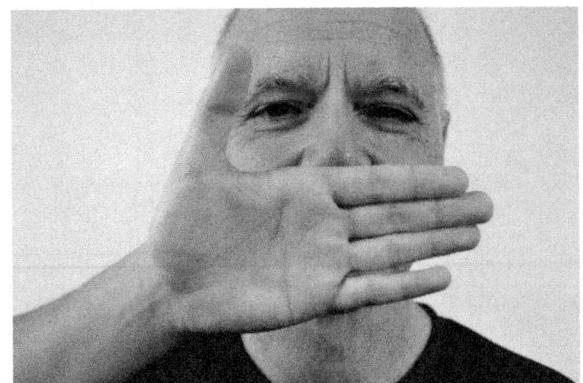

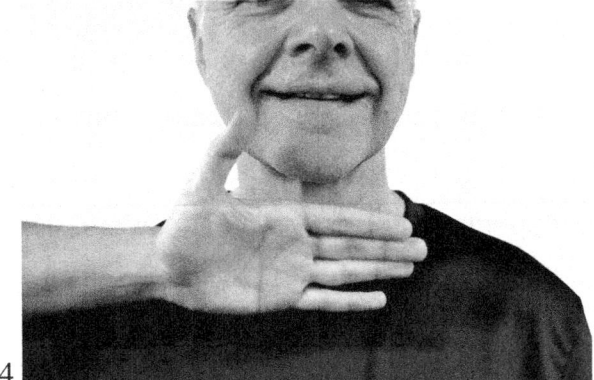

T-1

T-4

T-3

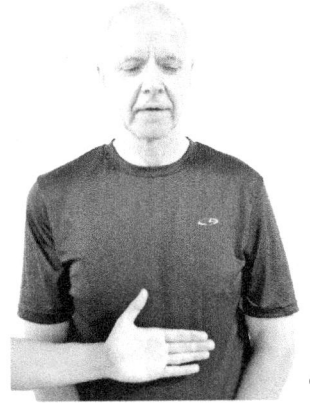

PRIMARY PHYSICAL POINTS

THYROID: The thyroid is broken down into three locations and you use your open hand – back and front - to test these points instead of your fingertips. You use the palm of your hand for the positive test, and the back of your hand for the negative. You don't actually touch the person when you test the thyroid, either; merely hold your hand a few inches in front of the point, first one side of the hand, then the other.

T-1 is the tip of the nose; hold your hand in front of the person's nose, (Palm first = Positive) and then back of the hand, (kNuckle – Negative), sort of like letting a dog sniff your hand before you try to pet it. T-1 blows only on children when they have thyroid problems.

T-4 is the front of the neck, at the base, where the thyroid gland is actually located. Again, use the front of your hand first, then the back of your hand, slightly in front of the person's neck.

T-3 is at the waist, or the belly button level. (Yes, T-3 is below T-4 …)

Is there a **T-2**? I have no idea! It's never mentioned!

BODY SPEAK

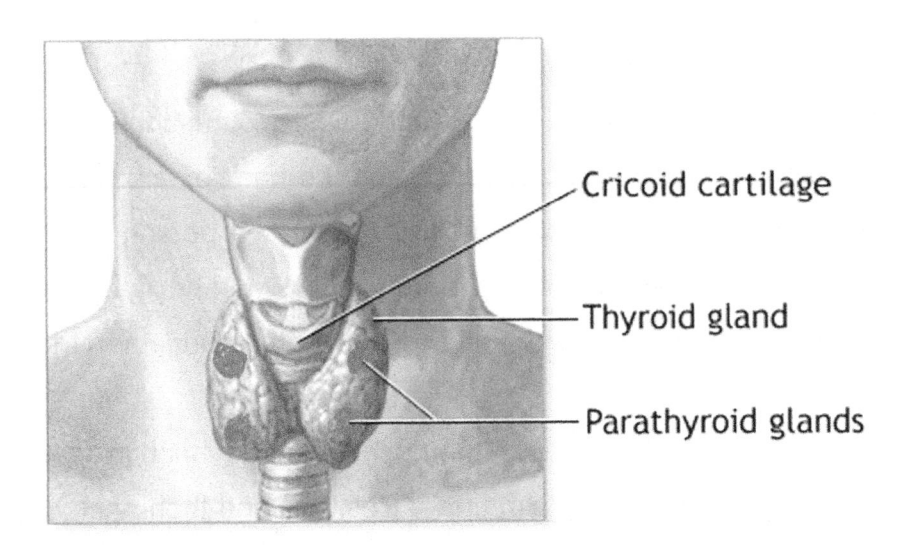

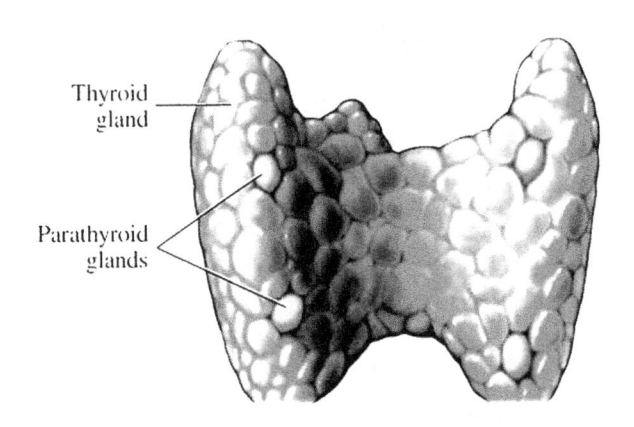

Back view of the parathyroid "buttons"

PRIMARY PHYSICAL POINTS

The **PARATHYROID** consists of four buttons, about the size of shirt collar buttons, on the thyroid gland, at the T-4 location. It often is a secondary point after thyroid T-4 and the hypothalamus have blown. This little, in size only, gland, when not functioning properly, can wreak havoc in the body and manifest in many, many ways, usually having to do with CALCIUM ASSIMILATION. Yes, here we go again. This is a "milkbox" for me, instead of a soapbox!

The four buttons are arranged in two rows of two, like a double-collared, button-down shirt, or in the four corners of a square, just below the Adam's apple. Test them individually. The top two buttons produce Vitamin F, and the bottom two produce Vitamin D. Both vitamins break down calcium and get the rather-large calcium molecules into and then out of EVERY CELL IN THE BODY. The tiny cells in the eyes and kidneys don't get calcium if the molecules are not broken down small enough and then we have eye or kidney problems. Calcium builds up like sludge in the intestines if it has not been broken down, used up, then carried away from the cells. The implications are vast and pervasive. Strength, energy, and calmness are the principle benefits of a well-

BODY SPEAK

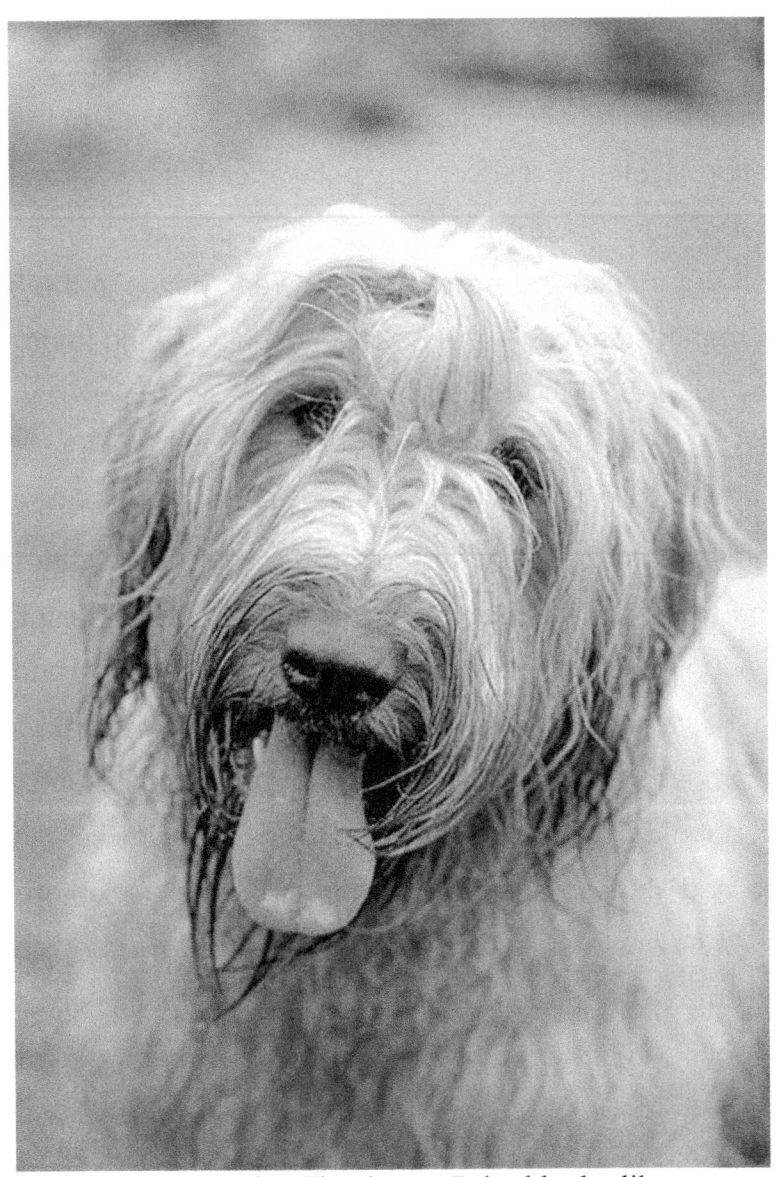

My sweet dog Shunka – a Briard look-alike

functioning parathyroid working with sufficient calcium. This is a very important point.

The parathyroid was the root cause of a problem a young man was having and I asked him if he had ever had his tonsils out, thinking that maybe the surgeon had nicked his parathyroid in the process. (Sometimes having a tube put down your throat will damage the parathyroid and/or the thyroid.) He said no, but that his little brother had tried to force a wooden arrow down his throat at one time. Bingo!

Cod liver oil is a great source of vitamin D, and flaxseed oil and safflower oil are great sources of vitamin F. I take two teaspoons of cod-liver oil and one teaspoons of flax oil regularly because of the history of osteoporosis in my family. Without these oils, my dog Shunka would not have been able to walk for the last several years of her life. She was a big dog and would have had hip dysplasia, but with the D and F, she was as limber and frisky as a puppy – until she stopped eating. The ratio for these oils, if both are needed, are usually cod liver oil 1:2 safflower oil or flax oil 1:2 cod liver oil. Be sure to dowse if one or both are needed, and how much.

BODY SPEAK

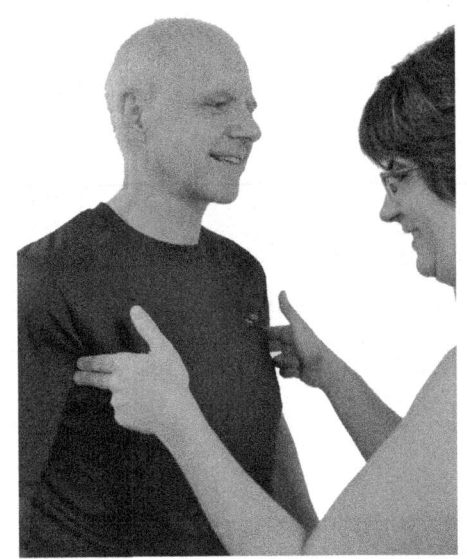

Adrenals testing points

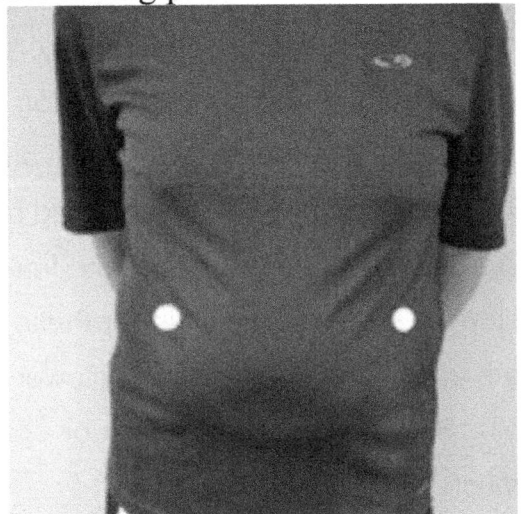

PRIMARY PHYSICAL POINTS

The two **ADRENAL GLANDS** are located on top of the kidneys and the test points for them are actually above and below the glands. Adrenals are tested at the armpits and just above the hips – four points.

Adrenaline is produced by the adrenal glands. Coffeeholics and people addicted to cocaine or methamphetamine have exhausted adrenals. Sometimes people with severe allergies who are forced to take strong antihistamines, in order to survive, have the same problem. Stress is another big factor in exhausted adrenals.

BODY SPEAK

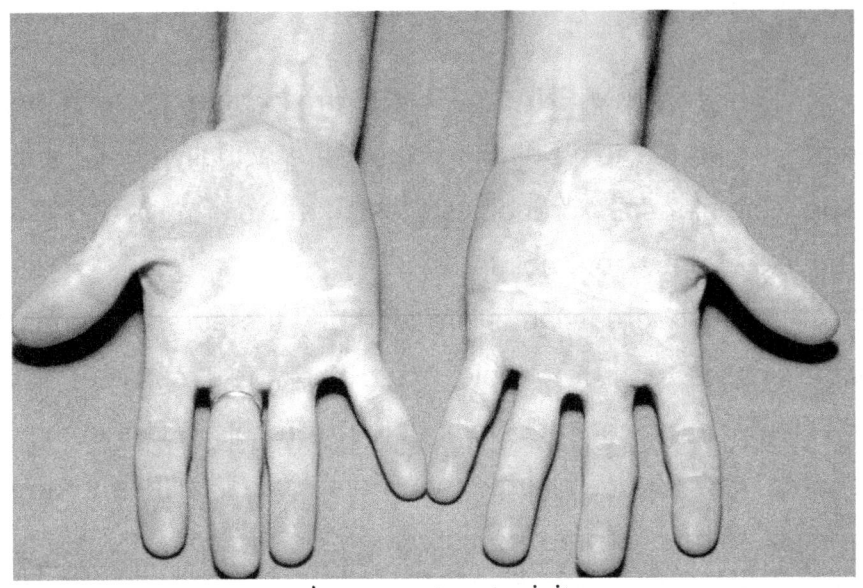

poison – system toxicity

PRIMARY PHYSICAL POINTS

POISON, System Toxicity: This point is the middle of the palms of the hands. If these points blow, notice the coloring of the palms. They will usually be an unhealthy red, getting darker and darker red at the fingertips, and the skin will be mottled. If you pinch a fingertip it will turn very white and then go back to the "angry" red. Detoxing with distilled water is a good remedy, as well as a good, cleansing diet for several weeks.[5] Processed food, particularly "fast food," loaded with salt, sugar, fat, preservatives and additives is a typical source of system poisoning.

---

[5] Dr. Andrew Weil, founder and director of the Andrew Weil Center for Integrative Medicine at the University of Arizona, has written 11 books on alternative health. I think they are all good. *8 Weeks To Optimum Health* is a great cleansing program.

BODY SPEAK

belly button

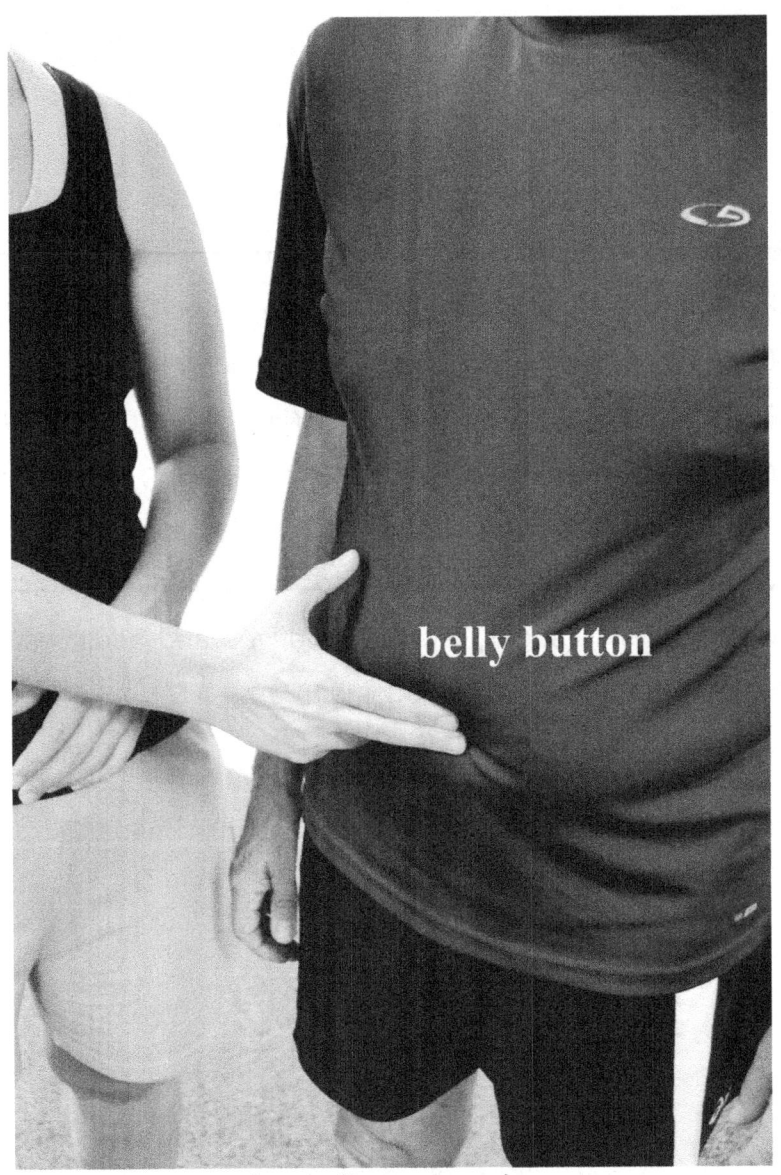

primary disease organisms

PRIMARY DISEASE ORGANISMS: This testing point is the belly button. The concept is simple, but I have had to ask a client occasionally where his belly button is because it was not obvious to me! One man had had an injury to his abdomen with subsequent surgery, and his belly button wound up quite a few inches left of center. I never would have found it without asking.

This point, **Primary Disease Organisms**, or **PDO**, is the point for testing for systemic diseases or infections caused by:

Bacteria	Mold – allergies, too
Fungus	Yeast.

Amoebae and parasites are also included in this list, and dysentery, usually contracted when traveling, is one of the illnesses caused by these foreign (literally) bugs.

If the PDO point blows, you must then test for the more specific problem to discover which type of PDO is causing the symptom. Keep asking until you have pinpointed the problem.

I tested a woman once who was very thin and whose symptoms were indigestion and regular bouts of diarrhea. She had been told that she had a spastic colon or colitis, I think. However, none of the regular cures had helped her at

BODY SPEAK

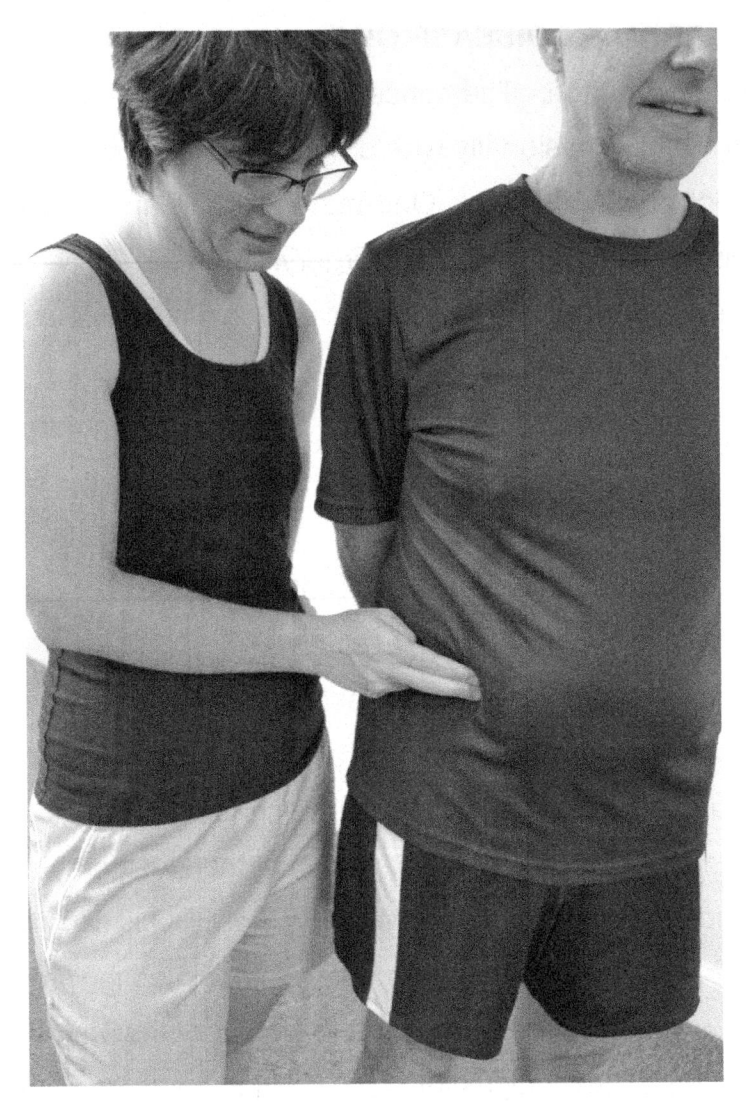

This point would cover the stomach and intestines when checking for parasites.

all. Drugs didn't work; diets didn't work. When I tested her, PDO was the root cause. After I rubbed it down, I tested her intestines and colon (see Chapter 3, as well) and they blew. I asked if it was parasites and got a very strong positive! It turned out that she had been a Peace Corps Volunteer some 20 years before, in a remote village and had never connected that adventure with her digestive problems.

    I first discovered HCl (hydrochloric acid) after suffering several severe bouts of dysentery one summer, working on an archaeological excavation in Turkey. The water was not potable, to say the least. My MD had prescribed a drug that, I found out later, stops peristalsis, the movement which the stomach and intestines make while digesting and processing your food. When there are foreign organisms in your gut, peristalsis goes into hyperdrive to try to get rid of the unwelcome guests, thus the diarrhea. If there is not enough hydrochloric acid to kill the parasites, the body will just keep trying to pump them out. And stopping the peristalsis without killing the organisms is only a 'stopgap' measure. The drug just attacks your autonomic nervous system and as soon as it wears off, the parasites start up again.

Peristalsis

- series of involuntary wave-like muscle contractions which move food along the digestive tract

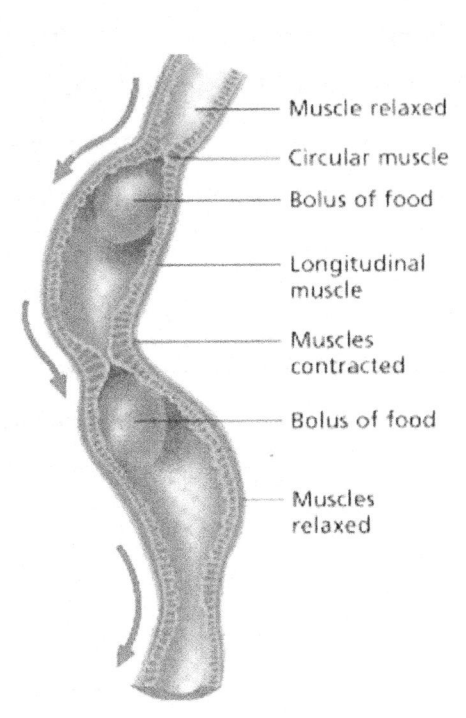

- Muscle relaxed
- Circular muscle
- Bolus of food
- Longitudinal muscle
- Muscles contracted
- Bolus of food
- Muscles relaxed

PRIMARY PHYSICAL POINTS

Hydrochloric acid is what we have in our stomachs to digest our food. So by boosting the acid, it kills the "turistas" and all is well. The increase in the amount of HCl cannot hurt unless one has a peptic (bleeding) ulcer. A doctor in San Francisco found that at least half of his patients who thought they had "acid stomachs" in fact did not have *enough* acid, and the symptoms were the same as if they had too much. We tend to have less in our stomachs as we get older, also. The HCl worked perfectly (one capsule with each meal) and my second summer in Turkey passed in great health. Everyone else got sick…

Health food stores carry HCl; and it usually contains betaine and/or pepsin, too, both digestive enzymes.

Then I discovered garlic. It got me through my third summer in Turkey with nary an unwelcome guest. It must be raw garlic, and it wants to be in pieces the size of a pill or capsule that you can comfortably swallow. Don't chop it up, and don't chew it up, either. You want it to stay whole through the digestive tract so it will kill the bugs wherever they are. It works just as well as the HCl, and is almost always available. People all over the world eat garlic and seem to know of its efficacy. If you dislike the taste of garlic or are afraid you will

BODY SPEAK

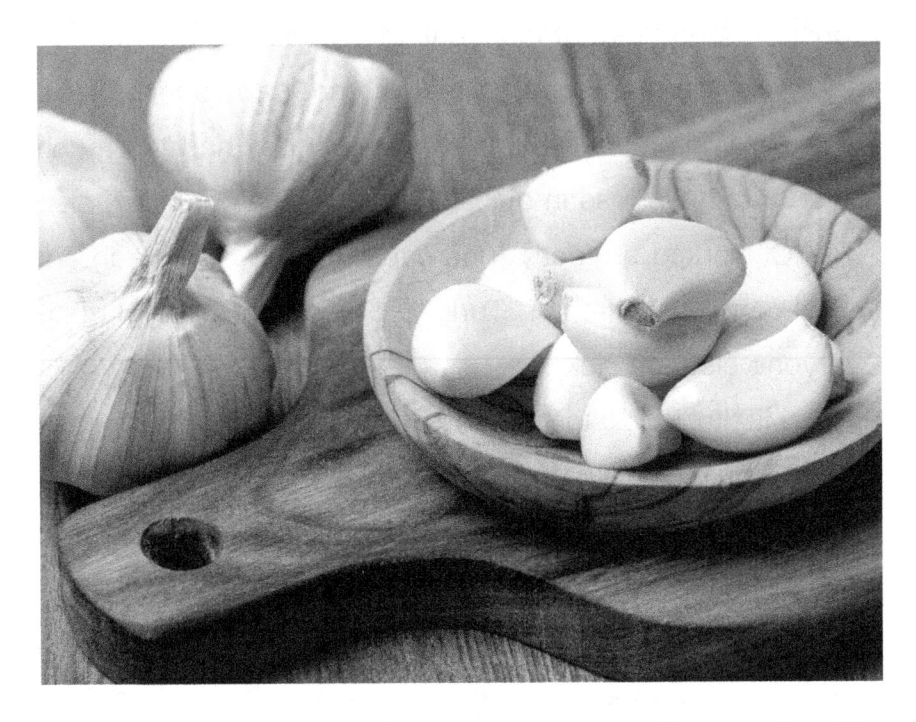

Cut a piece from a peeled clove that you can swallow comfortably.

smell of garlic, eat parsley, cilantro, or some dark, leafy greens. Chlorophyll is a deodorizer. Cooked garlic does not work and it would smell worse because the enzymes that digest the garlic have been killed.

Also, PLEASE NOTE: RAW GARLIC KILLS VIRUSES (like stomach flu) and CURES FOOD POISONING!!! Again, swallow a small piece or two and you will feel it going to work within minutes. There is no need to suffer. Garlic works.

Garlic also helps reduce cholesterol and blood pressure – another beneficial side effect.

If you look up natural remedies for parasites and amoebae, you will likely find a number of herbs including anise, black walnut, clove oil, diatomaceous earth, propolis, wormwood, and more. I know, from personal experience, that HCl (hydrochloric acid) with betaine and/or pepsin, and garlic, both work quickly and effectively.

BODY SPEAK

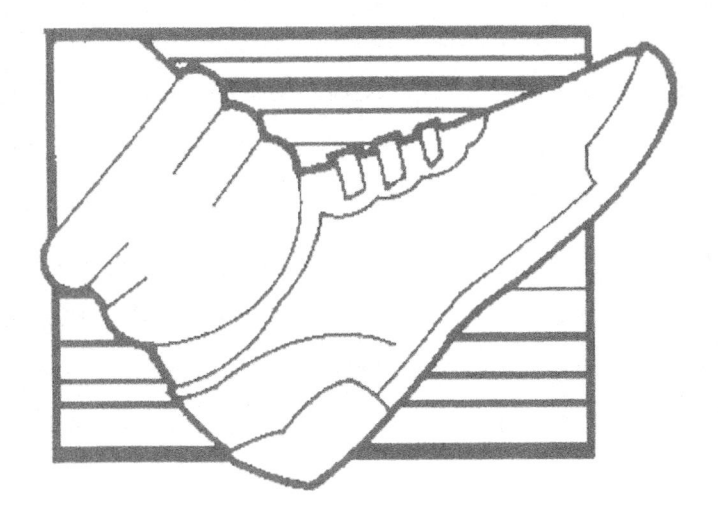

**Enclosed shoes,
made of synthetic materials
are a great breeding ground for fungus and yeast.**

PRIMARY PHYSICAL POINTS

More **Primary Disease Organisms**:

Athlete's foot is a common fungus, and thrives in damp, humid conditions. Go barefoot; wear shoes and socks made of natural materials; dry your feet really well after bathing. And you'll have no problem!

A carpenter/renovator friend of mine was [finally] diagnosed with an uncommon lung fungus carried by pigeon excreta that he had breathed in when working on various restoration projects. Fungal infections can be very serious and very difficult to get rid of especially when they are INSIDE our warm, water-logged bodies.

Chlamydia is a sexually-transmitted bacterial infection that has become more and more virulent and difficult to control. Women can get chlamydia in the cervix, rectum and throat. Men can get it in the penis, rectum and throat.

Candidiasis is a fungal infection caused by *overgrowth* of the **Candida** yeast which normally lives on the skin and inside the body of everyone. The upper left quadrant of a person's body is EXTREMELY sensitive if they have Candida. Once the PDO point has blown, a gentle touch in the area between breastbone and armpit and left shoulder and nipple will make a person with Candida wince and cringe.

Root Cause

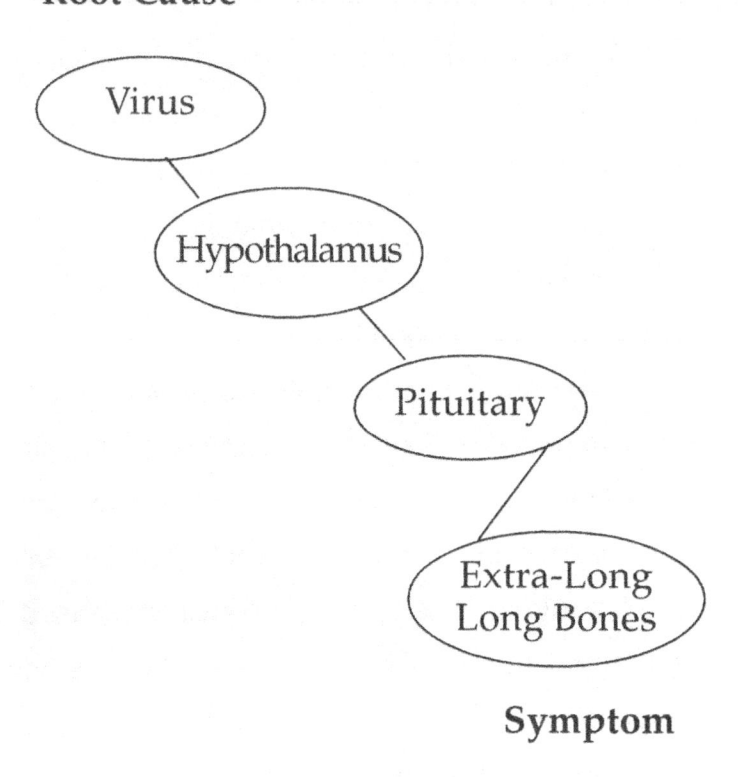

(Virus)

(Hypothalamus)

(Pituitary)

(Extra-Long Long Bones)

Symptom

PRIMARY PHYSICAL POINTS

VIRUS: The virus testing point is one inch below the belly button. If this point blows, rub it down and test again at the same point, because there are three sub-points, one of which will blow and that will give you a much better fix on the kind of virus it is:

1. If your fingers break on the first pull after you have discovered that a virus is the root cause, you will know that it is an ordinary current virus such as a cold, and will probably take one to two weeks to recover from. It will be of recent origin.

2. If your fingers break on the second pull, you will know that it is a very old, long-term virus; that the person has had the virus for a year or longer.

A favorite virus story comes from one of my husbands. Testing him for a certain symptom, the cause of the problem turned out to be a virus, which surprised me. And it blew again on the second pull, meaning a long-term virus; I had expected the hypothalamus or master brain. (And let me put in another warning here: *get rid of your expectations*. It can make your testing completely inaccurate. Sometimes I think a person does a much better job of testing when they don't know very much about human physiology or pathology!)

BODY SPEAK

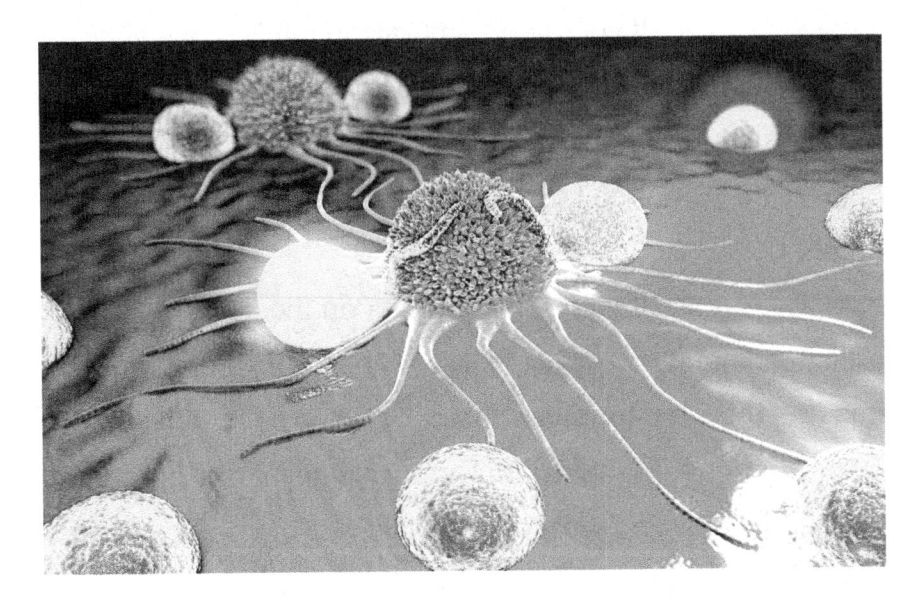

lung cancer cells

PRIMARY PHYSICAL POINTS

So after the virus point blew, I went back to the hypothalamus as a secondary point in this particular situation and sure enough, it blew. After asking various questions, it turned out that his mother had the exact same virus in her hypothalamus and passed it on to him in utero.

I don't mean to sound gleeful about any of my illustrations, but it is very satisfying, intellectually, to track down a root cause. I wonder if I have some not-so-secret desire to be a private eye?

Cancer is a virus, and if you work with this system for very long, you will definitely discover someone with cancer. I, personally, am not afraid of cancer and have no concern about it: forgiveness and dark leafy greens will cure cancer, especially with garlic sprinkled on liberally! I don't recommend telling anyone you have found cancer, however. Do think about how you might handle it. Supplements, a cleansing diet, and prayer work are a winning, healing, curing combination. Don't buy into doom and gloom! Remember, too, not everyone wants to heal; it might be subconscious, as it probably was for my mother. Many don't want to or don't know how to take responsibility for their own health. Our minds and thoughts control our health.

BODY SPEAK

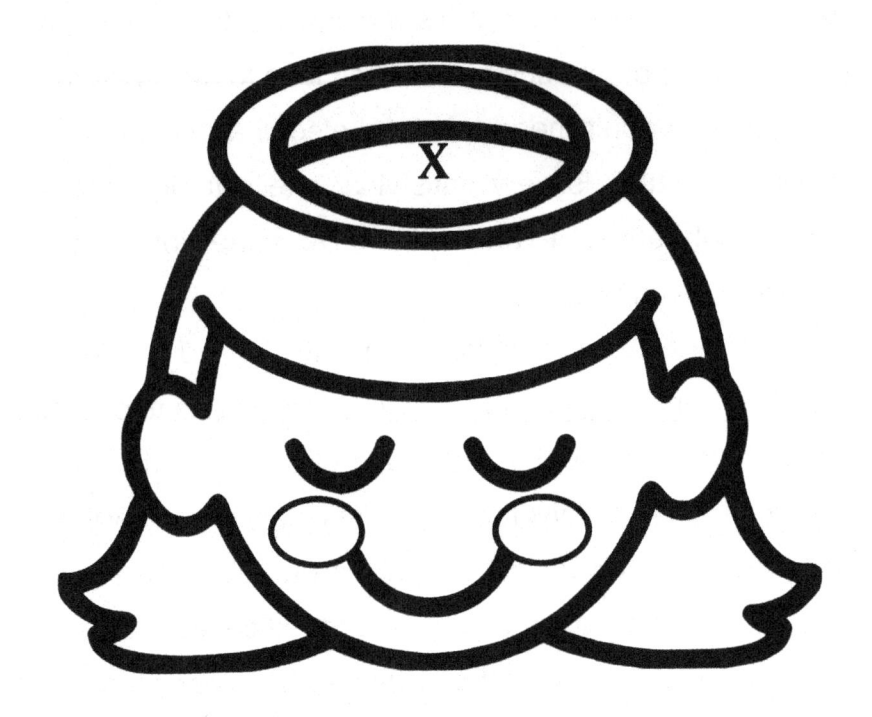

spiritual body point
above the head

PRIMARY PHYSICAL POINTS

If when you get to the end of this list you have not had even a slight weakening of your fingers anywhere along the line, try the

SPIRITUAL BODY point. This point is approximately four inches above the crown chakra, or the very top of the head. Imagine you or your client is wearing a halo: the spiritual body point would be the center of the halo! If this point blows, rub the point toward the back of the head and then go back to the physical body points, primary or secondary, until the chain of effect has been discovered and the symptom is the last point in the chain.

The spiritual body point can be the tip of a large and complex iceberg. The relief one can get from discovering and clearing the traumas that have been "frozen" in our spiritual bodies is as great as the iceberg. See Chapter 7.

BODY SPEAK

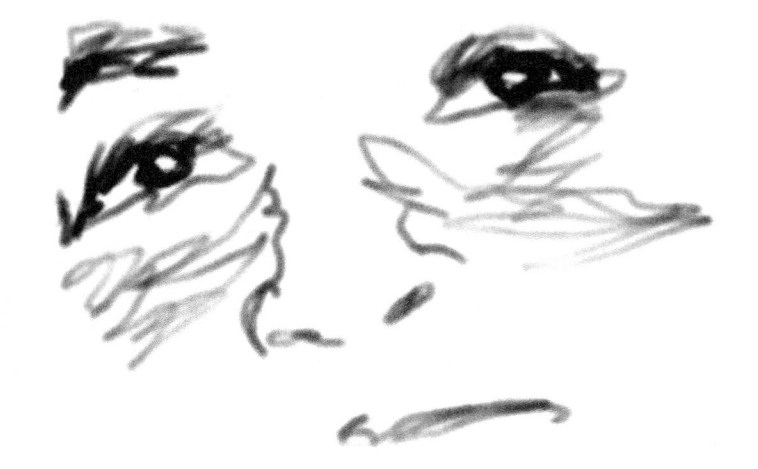

CHAPTER THREE
SECONDARY PHYSICAL POINTS

Naming this chapter "Secondary Physical Points" was an arbitrary decision. It is my experience that ANY POINT can be a primary point. What is the saying about rules being made to be broken? I mostly wanted to break down the points into more manageable pieces so you wouldn't go into overload – or commence snoring in the middle!

For example, the **EYES** can be the primary point if there has been damage directly to the eye. To test, place two fingers on the cheek bone right under the middle of the eye – for the irises – and at the outer corner for the eye as a whole. One of my sorority sisters was blind in one eye because her slightly older brother jabbed a pencil into it when she was an infant! Of course, she knew the cause of her blindness – that was no mystery – but it could certainly happen that a person have a trauma to an eye as a child and not remember it or not be able to communicate it if an adult did not witness the accident to tell the story later.

EARS: Place the two probe fingertips (one finger on top of the other) just into the ear to test for inner ear function, and the earlobe or bottom of the ear to check the outer ear.

BODY SPEAK

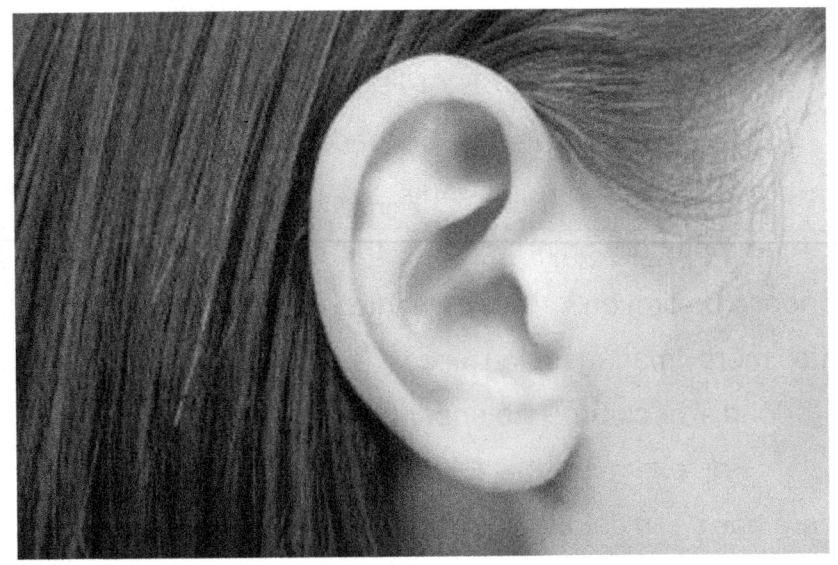

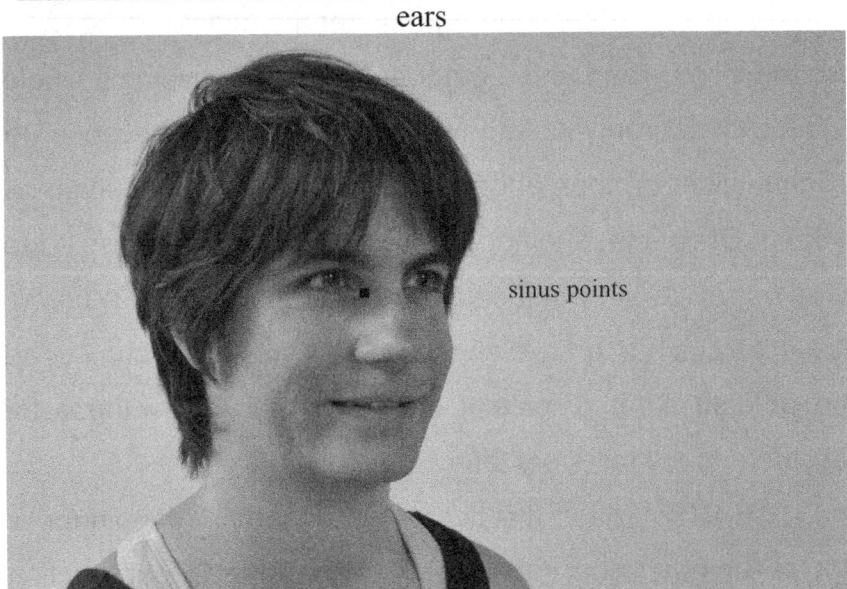

ears

sinus points

the inner corner of each eye
use index and middle fingers – straddling the nose

SECONDARY PHYSICAL POINTS

For hearing loss, place the hand flat over the ear, first the palm and then the back of the hand. If the positive (palm) test blows, the dysfunction is usually a long-term, old problem; if the negative (knuckle side) blows then the problem is usually acute – a recent infection or trauma.

When a child has an earache, 99.9% of the time it is a strep[tococcal] infection. The negative or knuckle side of the hand will blow – then check the point just under the child's jaw, a little back from the chin to confirm (or not) that it is a strep infection. [A small amount of warm vegetable oil with a few drops of garlic juice squeezed in will ease the pain and kill the infection.]

Tinnitus, which tends to show up in older people, is a degenerative disease of the body. In one person I tested, I found that a virus in the liver caused the pancreas not to function and the person's tinnitus was, essentially, a symptom of hypertension.

The **SINUS** points are the inner corners of the eyes and alongside the nose, and the forehead, brow line. Do furrowed brows come from sinus headaches?

BODY SPEAK

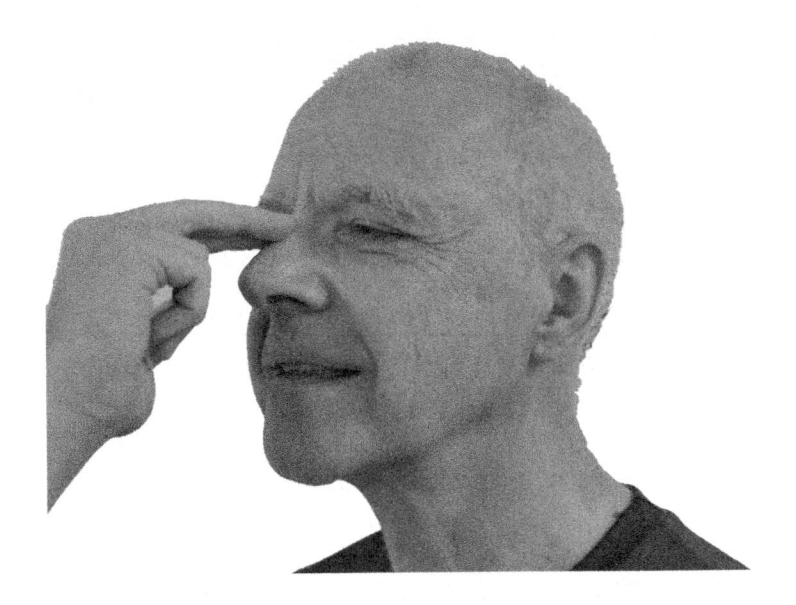

The hormones testing point is the same as the hypothalamus and the 'power point,' but you ask a different question.

SECONDARY PHYSICAL POINTS

HORMONES: The spot for hormone imbalance or dysfunction is the same spot as for the hypothalamus: the middle of the nose. When this spot is tested for hormones, however, you ask the person to give a regular pull – not the ten-second count as when testing the hypothalamus. See below (pages 118-121), the REPRODUCTIVE ORGANS, for the specific organs that are being affected by the hormone imbalance.

BODY SPEAK

Master Allergy point

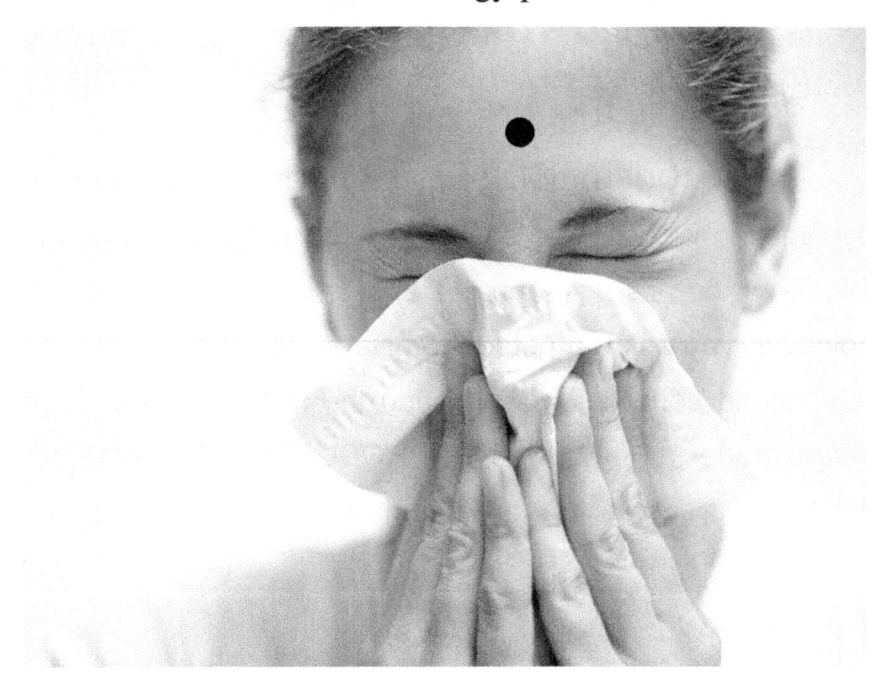

Allergies . . .

SECONDARY PHYSICAL POINTS

ALLERGIES: The Master Allergy point is in the middle of the forehead and if this point blows it means that there is an infection in the body. Rub down this point and then check the right and left points in order to narrow down the area of the infection.

The **Right** allergy point is the top of the right cheekbone, a finger's width away from the nose, and if this point blows it means the infection is in the right side of the body.

The **Left** allergy point is the top of the left cheekbone, a finger's width away from the nose, and if this point blows it means the infection is in the left side of the body. The left side of my body is the weaker – always has been. I have more problems with the teeth in the left side of my mouth; my left ear tends to have a continuous low-grade infection; when I have a cold, my left eye waters more and my nose runs more on the left side.

I cannot think of a time when I have been confronted with the need to know which side of a person's body an infection was present, but these points do remind me of the asymmetry of the body, so I am sure that one day the need for that knowledge will occur.

BODY SPEAK

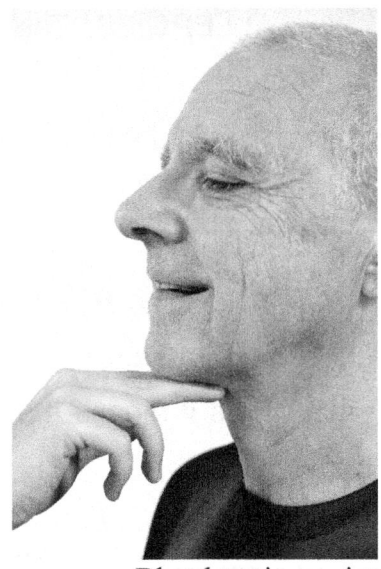

Blood testing point

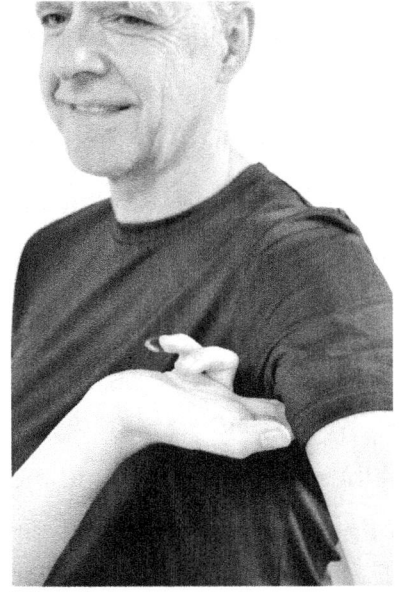

Blood pressure point

98

SECONDARY PHYSICAL POINTS

BLOOD: To test the blood point, use your open probe hand, first the palm side, then the knuckles side, under the chin. This point is above the T-4 point of the thyroid and can have to do with such problems as high cholesterol or leukemia.

The **BLOOD PRESSURE** point is the upper, inner, left arm, next to the lymph point if the arm were held close to the body. The "point" of this point is to verify that blood pressure is normal – or abnormally high or low. The root cause for any abnormality will come from any one of a myriad of causes. Use your two finger**tips** for low blood pressure, then turn your hand over and use the **nails** side of your fingers to test for high blood pressure.

BODY SPEAK

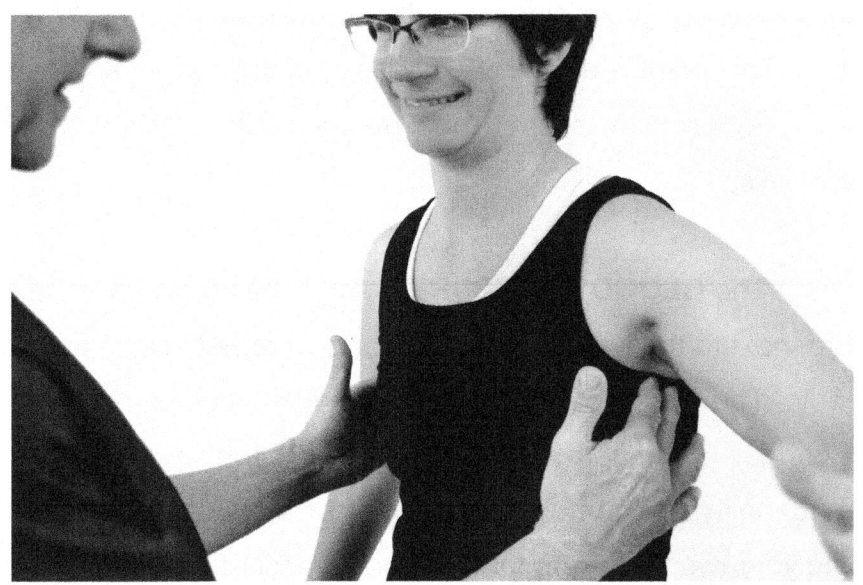

Lymph system

SECONDARY PHYSICAL POINTS

The **LYMPH SYSTEM** point is just into the armpit, behind the breast, on each side of the body. Lymph nodes are great cleaners of the blood along with the liver and the kidneys. We have probably all heard of a case of lymphoma cancer…

BODY SPEAK

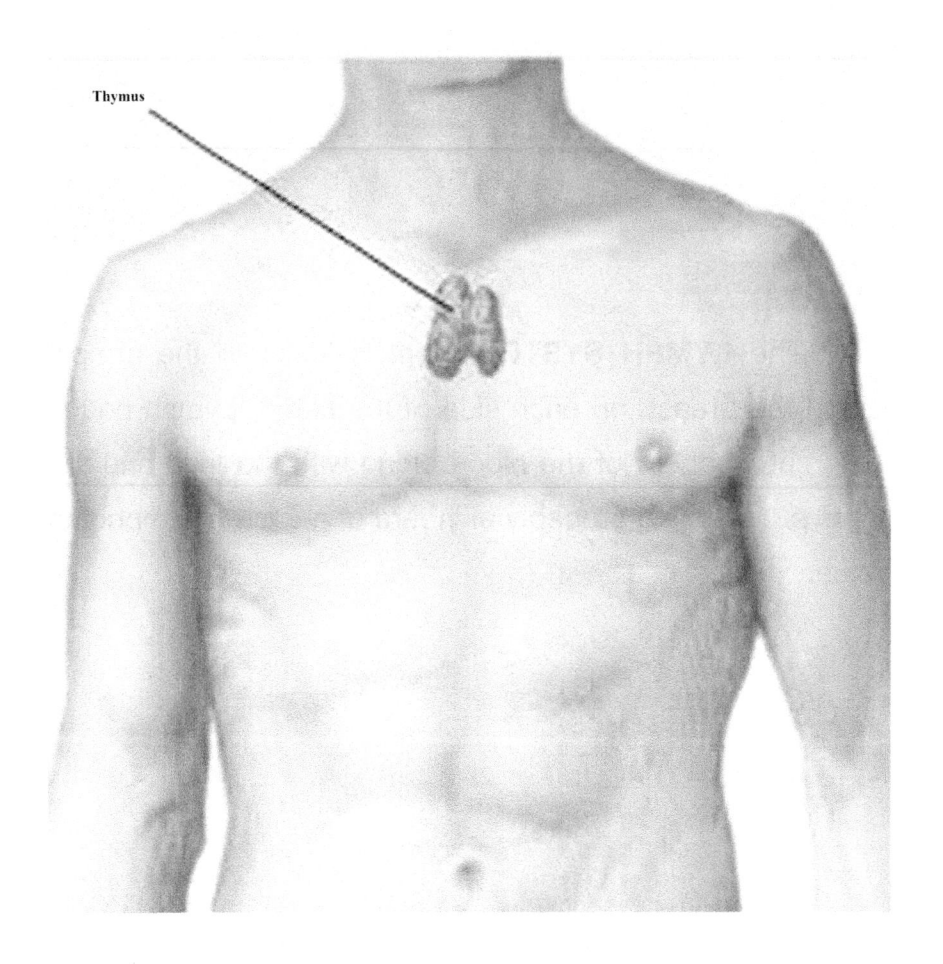

SECONDARY PHYSICAL POINTS

THYMUS: The thymus gland is located near the breastbone, on the left side of the chest, above the heart and about two inches below the notch in the collarbone. This gland is particularly important in early life in developing the immune system. You may be familiar with the name "sweetbreads" which is the thymus gland of young cows and is a very tasty dish if well prepared. Its importance in humans seems to diminish as a person matures, and atrophies somewhat later in life. If you feel yourself coming down with a cold or flu, thump (gently) with your knuckles on the thymus point for 2-3 minutes to stimulate your immune system.

This point might only be important in young people with a serious disease such as AIDS, but it could be a point in the "chain" of points in an adult with immune-system problems stemming from childhood trauma. There is a question, however, as to whether the thymus, like the appendix, actually serves a greater purpose that we are not yet aware of. I am not ready to "write off" either one yet!

BODY SPEAK

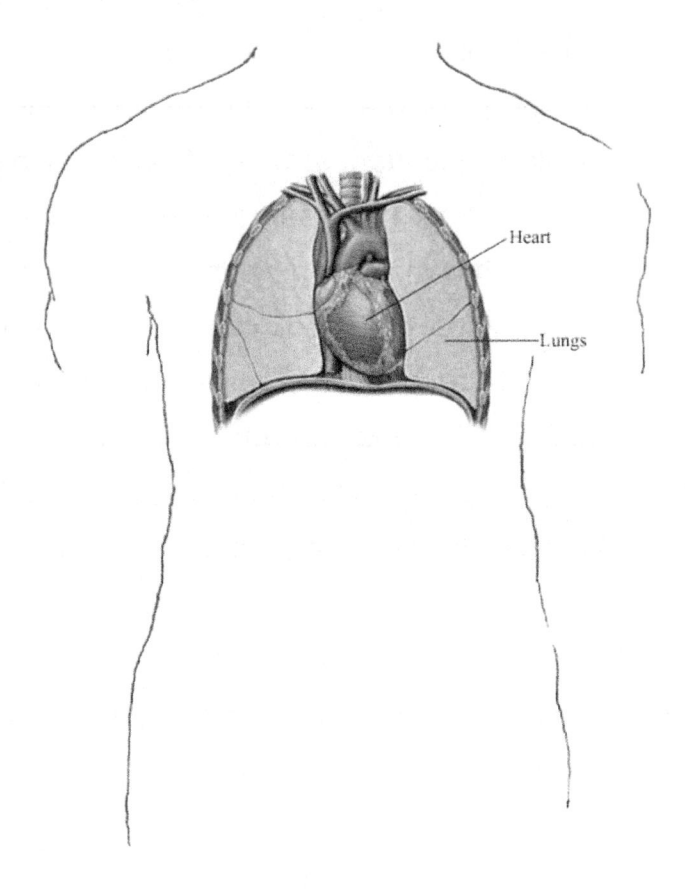

Heart and lungs

SECONDARY PHYSICAL POINTS

HEART: The heart point is just off-center to the person's left of the breastbone, and right of the nipple of his left breast (i.e., where the heart *is*). If the heart point blows, it can mean heart failure, arrhythmia, or a weak heart, or that the person is depressed or bloated (edema).

To test the **heart muscle**, ask the person to lock his thumbs together and extend his arms straight out in front of him (elbows straight) at shoulder height, as if he were going to dive. Test strength by pushing gently, but firmly down on the arms at the wrists.

LUNGS: The testing points for the lungs are both breasts, essentially, as the lungs extend from the collarbone to the diaphragm. They are usually secondary points to blow once it has been found that a virus or infection is the root cause of a symptom.

BODY SPEAK

Metabolic

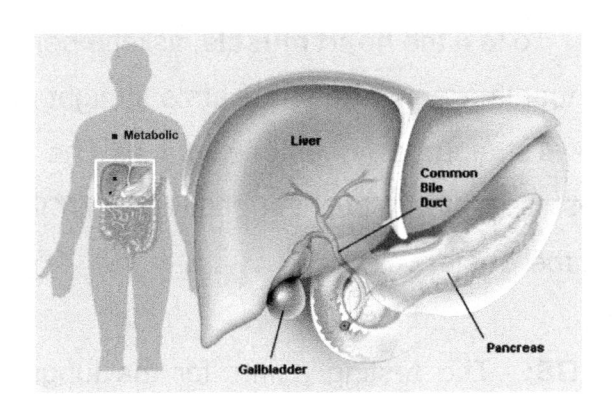

Liver   Gallbladder

SECONDARY PHYSICAL POINTS

METABOLIC: The metabolic point is in the [person's] right pectoral muscle, the middle of the quadrant whose boundaries are the top of the shoulder and the nipple, and the breastbone and the edge of the chest. This point has to do with how the body digests food, efficiently or not, and whether the body runs hot or cold.

LIVER: Under the right breast, and partly covered by the last of the rib cage is the liver point. The liver is very often involved with other organs as it sends hormones to the gall bladder, spleen and pancreas, for starters, and is extremely important to the health of the body because of its filtering and toxin-removing functions. Severe alcoholics die of cirrhosis of the liver when their livers cannot cope any longer with the large amounts of alcohol being consumed. The different types of hepatitis are all liver dysfunctions. Jaundice is another form of the liver being overloaded with toxins to process.

The **GALL BLADDER** is between the liver and the spleen, just under the stomach. Its function is very important in the digestion of fats.

BODY SPEAK

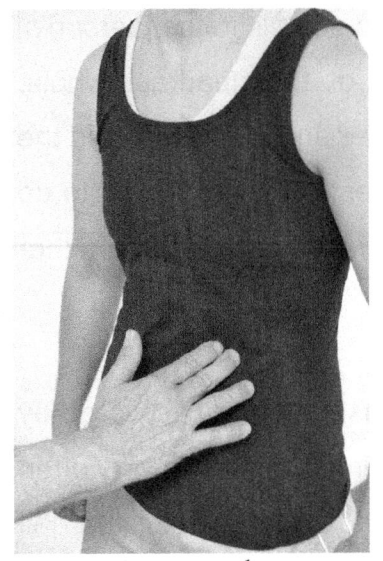

stomach

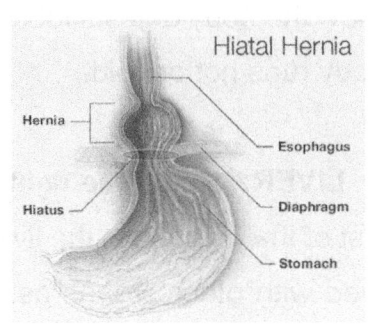

hiatal hernia

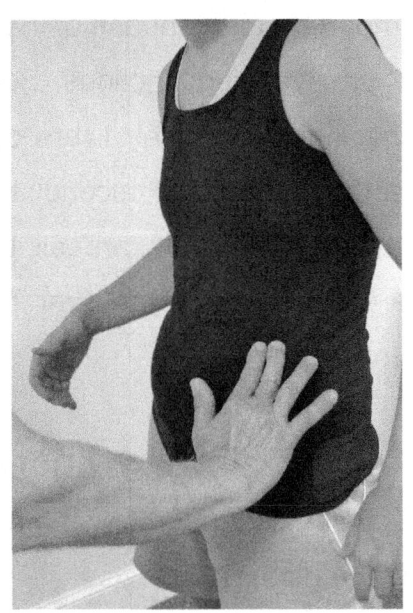

spleen

SECONDARY PHYSICAL POINTS

The **STOMACH** point is down from the left breast, at the bottom of the rib cage, in the center of the abdomen.

The **HIATAL HERNIA** point is the left part of the diaphragm. A hernia is an organ or part (of an intestine, for example) that pushes through the muscle or tissue that encloses it. A hiatal hernia is a bulge from the end of the esophagus where it empties into the stomach. Other hernias are esophageal hernias (at the top end of the esophagus, or the throat), belly button hernias which babies sometimes have (sometimes from being jerked up by their feet too roughly when they are delivered), or which adults can have from severe coughing.

Hernias can sometimes be relieved by manipulation – and then a good diet. Plenty of Vitamin C strengthens the cell wall structure which, in turn, can heal the hernia or the break in the peritoneum.

SPLEEN: The spleen is located under the left breast, below the rib cage, just to the right of the stomach as you are looking at the person. Multiple Sclerosis patients usually have spleen infections.

BODY SPEAK

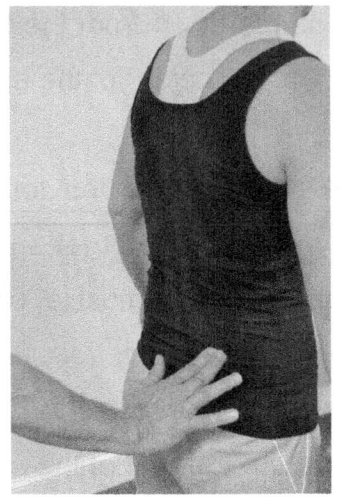

right kidney

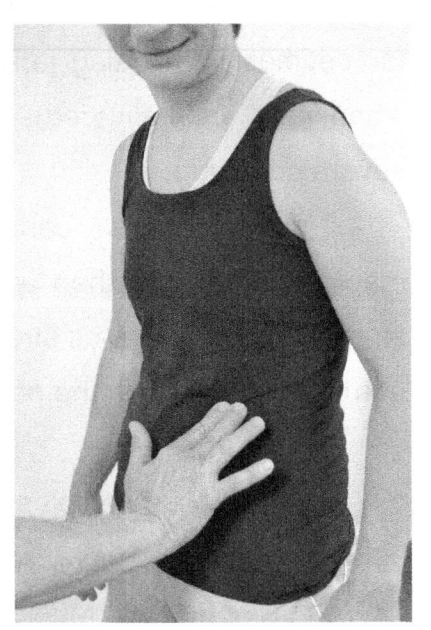

pancreas

SECONDARY PHYSICAL POINTS

KIDNEYS: One inch above the navel, and with two fingers spread (creating a V), one inch on either side of the navel is the testing point **from the front** – or, if you are standing **facing the person's back,** point your "forked" fingers at the waistline. You can also use two fingertips to touch each side, but you don't have to touch the person for this point; your intention is to test the kidneys.

The **PANCREAS** is located just to the right of the spleen, looking at the person, at the edge of the abdomen before it goes "around the corner." The pancreas is the organ that produces insulin which breaks down sugar. In the case of diabetes, the pancreas cannot produce enough insulin to process sugar that is ingested. Incidence of pancreatic cancer has increased exponentially in recent years.

BODY SPEAK

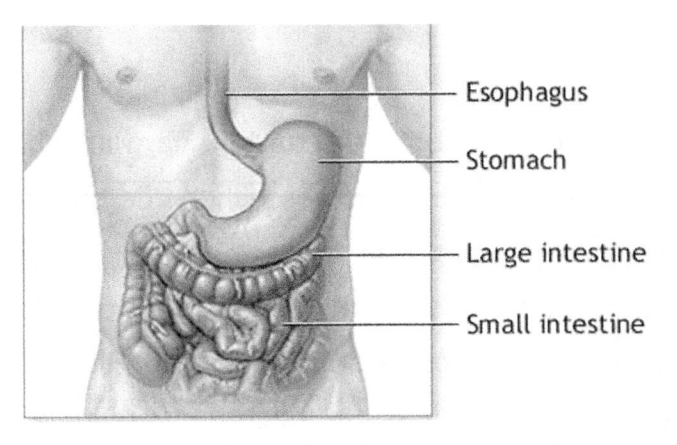

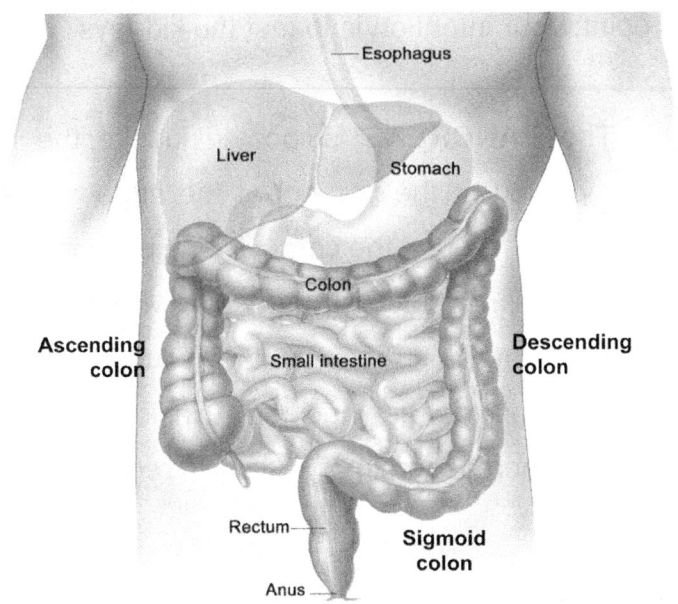

SECONDARY PHYSICAL POINTS

INTESTINES and **COLON:** The "package" of the intestines and colon is like a square, with the small intestines inside the square – the top half, the large intestines also inside the square – the lower half, and the colon describes the square.

When you come upon hot spots in this part of the body, it can indicate the location of parasites, diverticulosis and/or diverticulitis. Diverticulosis is the condition of protruding pockets developing along the intestines. These can come from calcium buildup, severe flatulence (from the lack of flora and fauna in the intestines from taking drugs or eating processed foods, partially digested food getting "stuck," not being able to move through the rest of the digestive tract., etc. Diverticulitis is when these pockets get infected; it then becomes a much more serious issue. Clues to the cause of one of these points blowing should come from the primary points that have blown before them.

BODY SPEAK

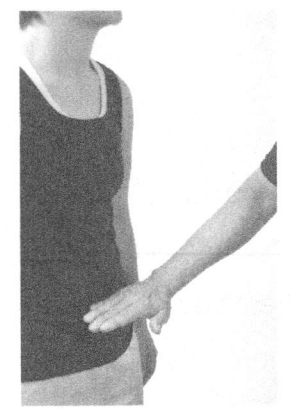

small intestines

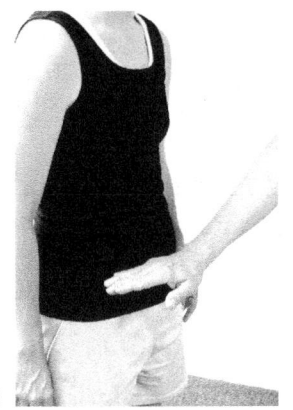

large intestines

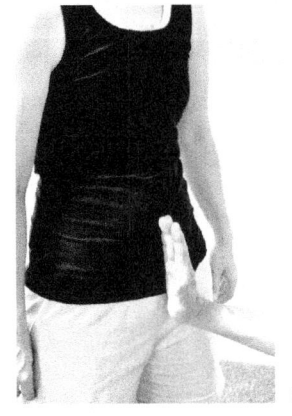

colon

SECONDARY PHYSICAL POINTS

To test the intestines, use the side of your probe hand as if you were going to karate-chop the person. Look at the photos on the opposite page. The small intestines are closer to the belly button; the large intestines below. The colon "starts" with the ascending colon, on Audrey's right side. (The picture on the opposite page, however, shows the descending colon being tested which is on the person's left side.) After testing the small, then large intestines, test the ascending colon holding your hand vertically, fingers up, on the person's right side. Then test the transverse colon, your hand parallel to the floor, just above the small intestine point. See page 112. Test the descending colon (the last picture on the opposite page) and then the Sigmoid colon, which is about half of the bottom of the square, the right half (as you face your client). The sigmoid colon empties into the rectum and then goes out of your body through the anus.

BODY SPEAK

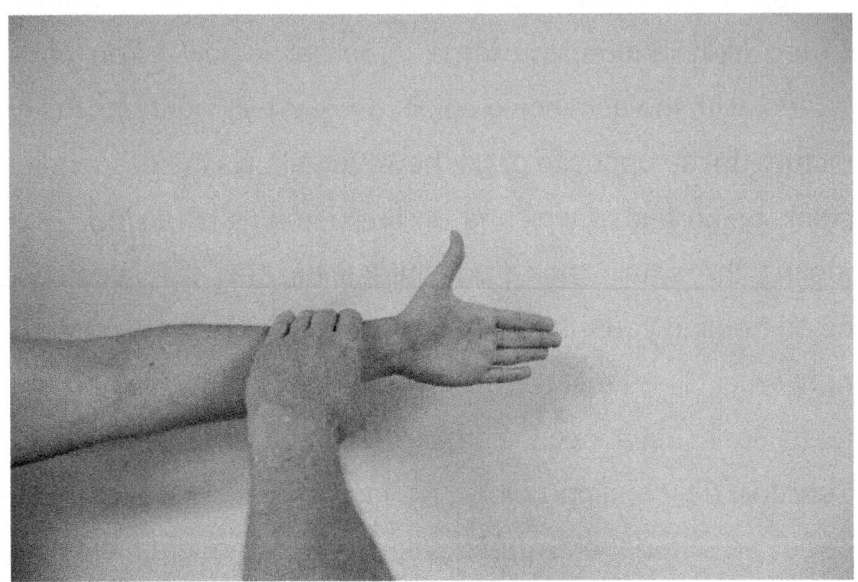

bone testing point

SECONDARY PHYSICAL POINTS

BONE: I usually use the wrist, or a little below, onto the forearm, for this point. The arm is one of the sets of long bone, and the wrist is a *handy* joint to test. (One of my congenital defects is my sense of humor which means, in my family, lots of puns and "bad" jokes. I'm sure you have figured that out by now. My dad was one of the best – or worst, depending on your perspective, punsters I have ever known.) This point can have to do with growth (or lack of growth) of the long bones; often in combination with the pituitary.

CALCIUM (various): For these points, I use the chiropractic method of muscle resistance (the client extends his arms and I push down on them with my hands, as I face the person, and see if they can resist my pressure). The person being tested extends both his arms straight out from the shoulders to his sides, hands open and flat, fingers extended. The four points being tested are:

BODY SPEAK

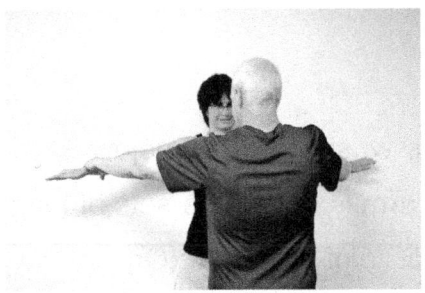

thumbs forward: calcium deficiency

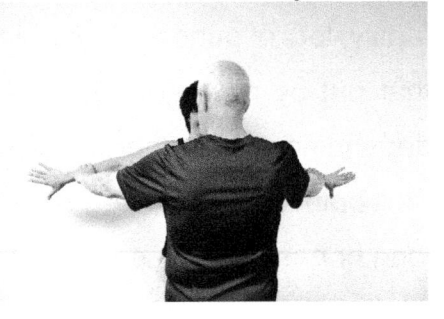

thumbs down: osteoporosis

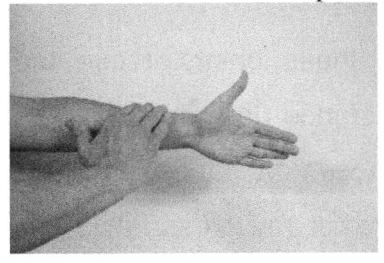

thumbs up: gout / arthritis

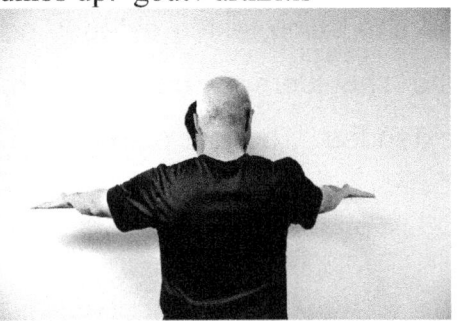

thumbs back: slipped disc

SECONDARY PHYSICAL POINTS

When the (1.) <u>thumbs are forward</u> and the arms are weak, it signifies that the person has a **calcium deficiency**. This is in contrast to the body just not assimilating calcium (when the parathyroid is not functioning to full capacity, for example), and means that more calcium needs to be taken in, ideally from fruits and vegetables.

If the person cannot resist your pressure when his (2.) <u>thumbs are down</u> (the backs of his hands are facing you), it means the person has **osteoporosis**. You can then check for the specific locations of where the osteoporosis is manifesting.

When the (3.) <u>thumbs are up</u>, open palms facing you, it means that the person has **gout** or **arthritis**. The kidneys will be sore to the touch, also, as gout usually comes from a severe staphylococcus infection of the kidneys. (People with gout should stay away from beef, turkey and wheat, by the way.)

If the person cannot resist your pressure while the (4.) <u>thumbs are back</u> (palms up), it means that there is a **slipped disc** (in the spine) or a disc that is **ruptured** or **degenerating**.

BODY SPEAK

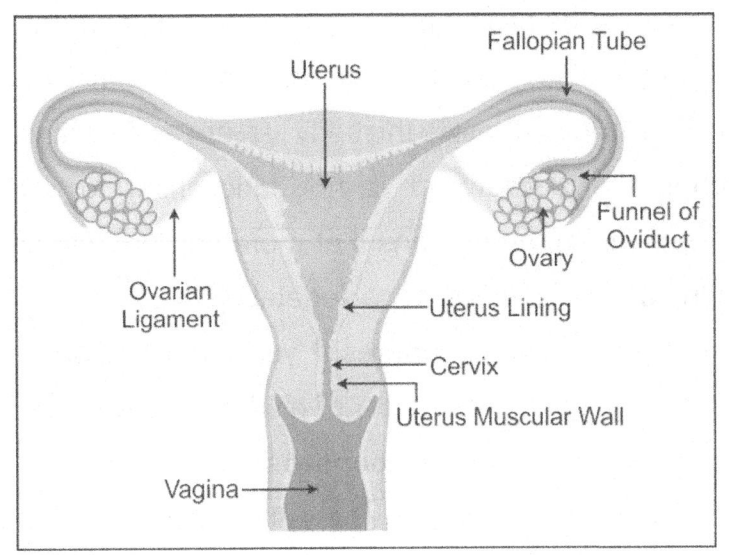

female reproductive system

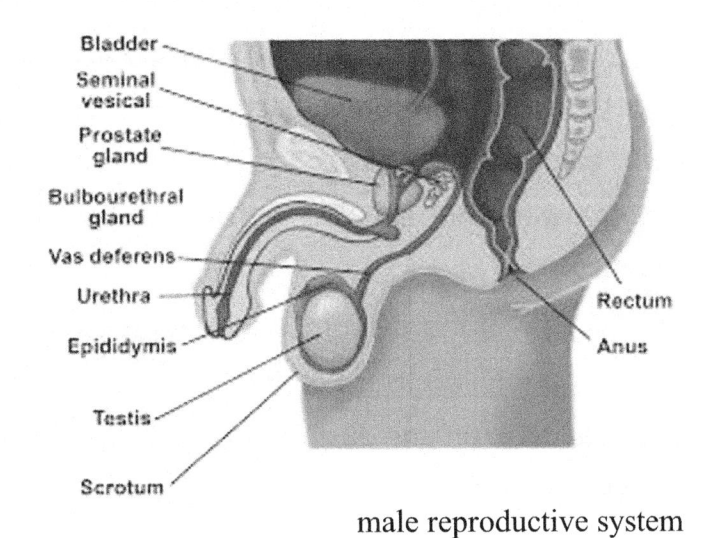

male reproductive system

SECONDARY PHYSICAL POINTS

The **REPRODUCTIVE ORGANS**, or points for testing the organs, are most likely NOT going to be primary points. Infection or virus will probably be primary points, then the reproductive glands will blow as secondary points in the chain. The possible problems are myriad as are the sources of the problems.

I have been very interested in this part of our physiology probably because I had so many problems before I finally had the wonderful, trouble-free pregnancy with my daughter. I spent years in gynecologists' offices, in compromising positions, trying find out why I wasn't getting pregnant – and subsequently – why I wasn't staying pregnant. Dr. King opened my eyes and my mind to the world of medicine from the perspective of an OB/GYN specialist. But he had practiced medicine long enough that he knew drugs and surgery did not work, long term. If he or I had been a dowser back then we would have discovered that I had a serious hormone imbalance. Whether he knew specifically that I had a hormone imbalance or that staying away from sodium-based animal protein would give my body a boost and restore balance, I don't know. But it worked. And I discovered much later why the vegetarian diet worked so well for *me*.

BODY SPEAK

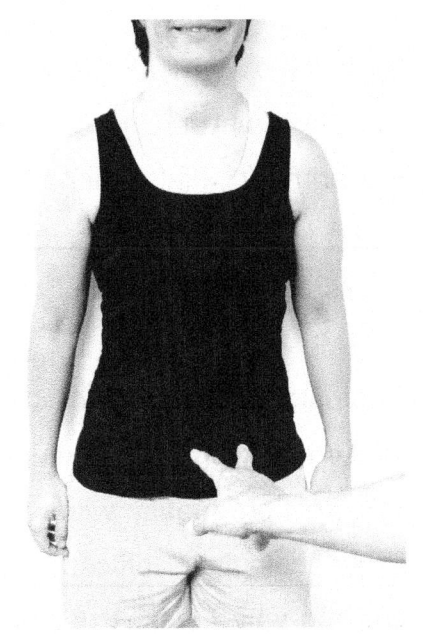

ovaries

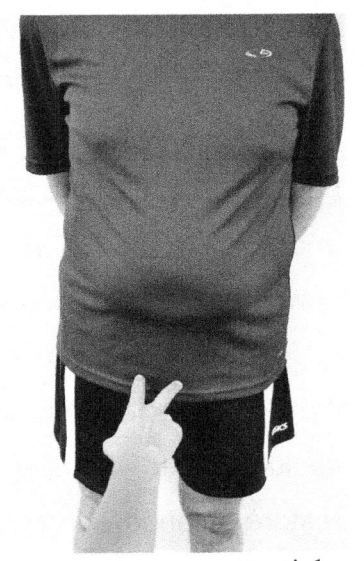

testicles

SECONDARY PHYSICAL POINTS

I wanted my daughter so much and she has been so incredibly special to me that I feel particularly empathetic to those who want to have children and have found the path fraught with obstacles and barriers. I cannot imagine my life not being a mother – and I am grateful that I don't have to live it childless. Since my education is in sculpture, I firmly believe that my daughter is the most creative "sculpture" I ever made! And she's kinetic!

OVARIES: Separate your two probe fingers and "aim" them at points just below and on either side of the navel.

FALLOPIAN TUBES: Separate your two probe fingers as in testing for the ovaries, but point your fingers down, the back of your hand being closest to the woman's abdomen and your wrist being about navel level.

TESTICLES: Separate your two probe fingers slightly, and "aim" them at the base of the pelvic area, at the top of the legs, where the testicles would be.

The **PROSTATE** gland is located at the base of the urethra and is partly muscle, partly gland. It secretes an alkaline fluid which carries the sperm in an ejaculation. It is this gland that has been a cancer spot for so many men in the last 30 years.

BODY SPEAK

I feeeel good . . . . (ta duh ta duh ta duh ta duh . . . .)

I knew that I would now . . . .
                                                  James Brown

SECONDARY PHYSICAL POINTS

The **URETHRA** is the tube, in men and in women, that is the conduit for urine from the bladder out of the body. In women, the end of the urethra is an opening just above the vaginal opening; and in men, the urethra runs the length of the penis and is the conduit for both urine and seminal fluid when ejaculation occurs.

BREASTS: Any point on the breast can be tested if that is your intent – and don't forget men can have breast problems as well as women.

The stories are endless – and to me, at least, fascinating:

A medical technologist who worked for many years in hospital nurseries told me 25 years ago, that one out of four newborns were androgynous = neither male nor female, no sex [not hermaphrodites = both sexes]. The implications are mind boggling.

BODY SPEAK

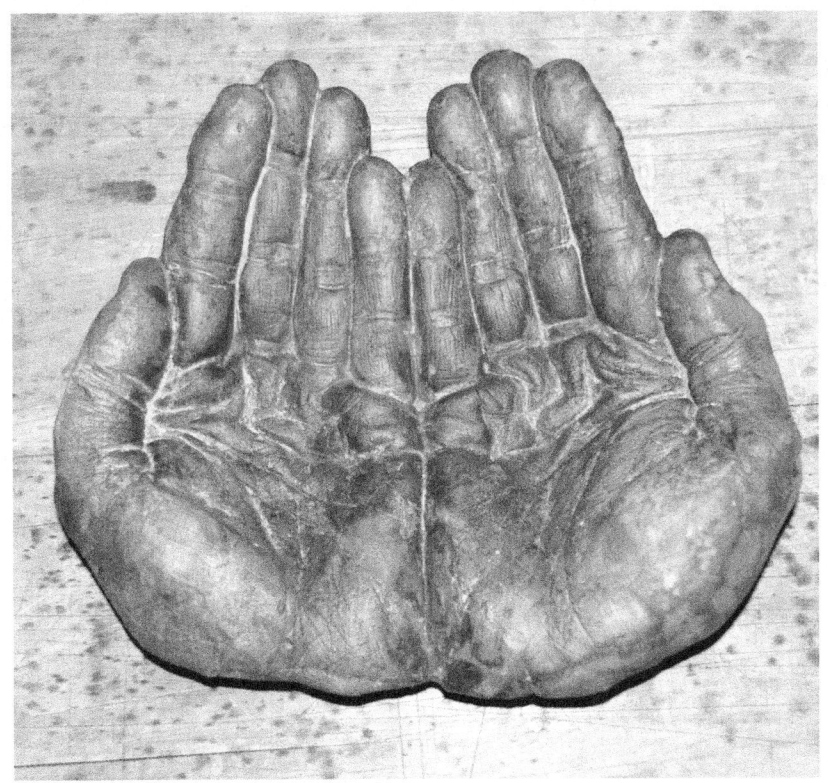

My non-sexist rationale: I like to think we are called
hu-mans because we have *mains* / *manos* = hands =
fingers with an opposing thumb
so that we can *mani*pulate things.
(But the etymology does not bear me out!)

SECONDARY PHYSICAL POINTS

There is a large segment of our population that is homosexually oriented and/or desires to change their sex.

The "insecticides" that are being used now in American agribusiness in fact do not kill insects, but rather keep insects from being able to reproduce. These chemicals are an estrogen-like chemical which we, in turn, ingest and then have all kinds of problems with *our* reproductive organs. I am less knowledgeable about the effects on men, but women being inundated with so much estrogen results in many that are not able to produce enough progesterone to keep their systems in balance to have healthy pregnancies, so they have miscarriages and spontaneous abortions; they get breast cancer, ovarian cancer, migraines, PMS, osteoporosis. Twenty-three (now 43) years ago, I became a vegetarian so that I could have a better shot at getting pregnant, staying pregnant and having a healthy pregnancy and child. It worked beautifully; not eating meat encouraged my own hormones to work properly without the burden of steroids and other chemicals fed to animals raised for meat. And the insecticides then were not based on hormones, so my body was able to produce enough progesterone to "stay pregnant." It was

BODY SPEAK

Indian Chole with Lemon Rice

3 c. cooked garbanzo beans (or the right kind for your blood type!)
    Make a puree of the following (or don't) of
    1 walnut-sized ball of tamarind, softened
    1 c. diced red onion
    3 cloves of garlic, halved
    1 T. minced ginger root
    1 T. molasses
    2-1/4 t. cinnamon
    1-1/4 t. salt (I never use salt when I cook)
    1-1/2 t. ground coriander
    1-1/4 t. ground cumin
    1 t. paprika
    8 black peppercorns (or ground black pepper)
    ½ t. turmeric
    ½ t. ground cardamom
Heat
    1 T. vegetable oil and add
    2 dried red chiles
then add the above spices/puree (with some of the bean liquid) and after a few minutes add:
    3 c. water or vegetable stock (or less)
    1-1/2 c. chopped tomatoes (may use canned)
    1 c. diced carrots (or yams/sweet potatoes)
    1 c. diced potatoes
    1 c. chopped cabbage
    2 minced Serrano peppers (optional)
    3 T. chopped mint (or 1 t. dried peppermint or contents of a peppermint teabag)
    2 t. cumin seeds
and cook awhile or until you can't stand the good smells anymore!

Serve over Lemon Rice (lemon zest in Basmati rice).

actually only a few years ago that I suddenly realized that my taking "the pill" for six years in my early twenties, seemingly without side effects then, had been at least partly to blame for throwing my hormones completely off balance, making the production of progesterone in my body insufficient to counteract the "overdose" of estrogen and thus not allowing the egg to attach to the wall of my uterus once I did conceive.[6] Becoming a vegetarian allowed my hormones to get back into balance and produce what was needed for a health pregnancy without having to fight against the estrogen in commercially-raised meat or the consequences of taking a birth control pill. That was then, however. The estrogen-like "pesticides" that keep insects from being able to reproduce and the estrogen-like molecules that are off-gassed from new plastics are inescapable in our modern society. No wonder we are having so much trouble having babies: getting pregnant – and staying pregnant to full term. Once again, we can't produce enough progesterone to maintain the necessary balance for a healthy, full-term pregnancy and a healthy child.

---

[6] Dr. John R. Lee, *Natural Progesterone.* This is a factual and definitive book about why women's hormones are out of balance – AND how to fix the situation.

BODY SPEAK

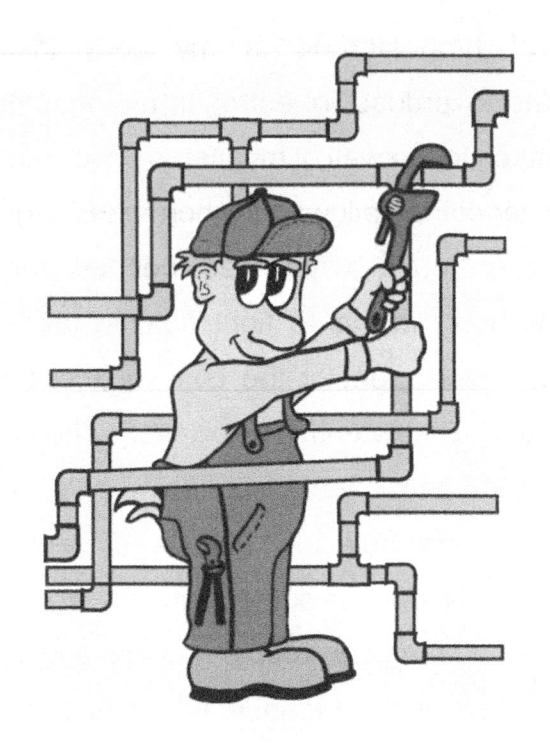

It's usually a matter of plumbing!

SECONDARY PHYSICAL POINTS

About ten years ago, I discovered another reason why becoming a vegetarian was so beneficial for me. I believe this "therapy" is of huge importance to us all. See Chapter 5!

Even though I know, after writing about estrogen overdose being a major cause of reproductive problems, I still feel that there are too many women getting breast cancer, and too many men getting prostate cancer. And I would like to know why. Is it a race-consciousness problem? Is this how overpopulation is going to cure itself and we are going to get back into a manageable population – by drastic reduction of birthrate by no-sex people, homosexual people and people who die with a reproductive organ disease who have never had children? The questions are terrible and fascinating to me and I have a way of getting answers. I love being a dowser and I am extremely grateful to Spirit for this gift. I'm not always happy with the answers, however.

The last chapters, 6 – 8, present some other possible answers to questions of causes of illness.

BODY SPEAK

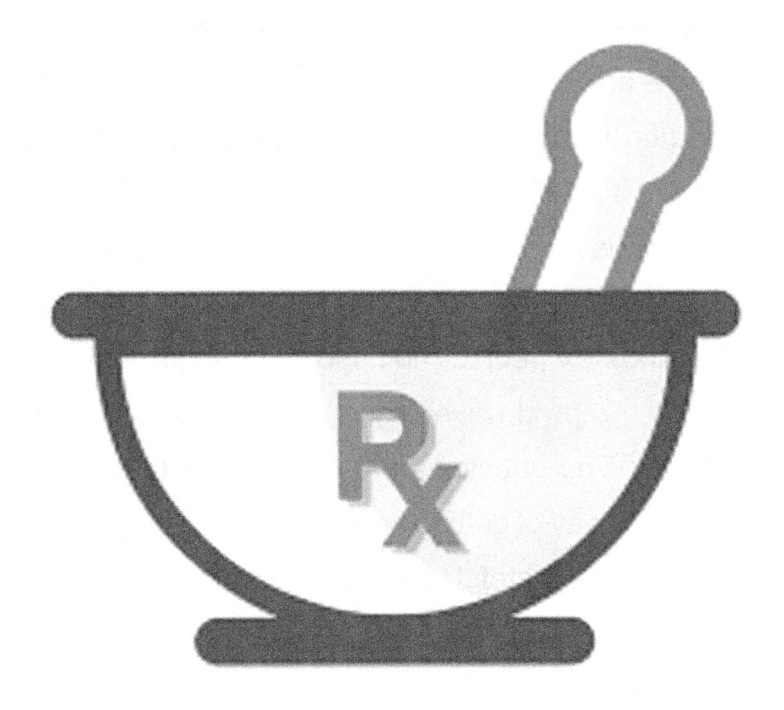

CHAPTER FOUR
REMEDIES

But let's look at some remedies! Now that you have a nice, neat diagram of the root cause and the subsequent links in the chain of hot spots leading from it to the symptom, what next? There are many possibilities and here are some that I can suggest: 1) nutritional/ herbal/glandular extract remedies, 2) magnet or crystal broadcasting, and/or 3) clearing.

When I learned this muscle testing from Sarah Meredith, I was coming from a long history of interest in nutrition. I had read lots of books on nutrition, health foods and diet and so I fell right into using nutritional remedies such as vitamins, minerals, some herbal remedies and glandular extracts about which Sarah was also teaching us. Sarah had had two years of chiropractic studies plus growing up with a father who was a chiropractor.

We worked with companies such as Standard Process and Nutri-West and used their product lists as charts to dowse for nutritional help in supporting the organs and glands that were dysfunctional. Standard Process and Nutri - West

BODY SPEAK

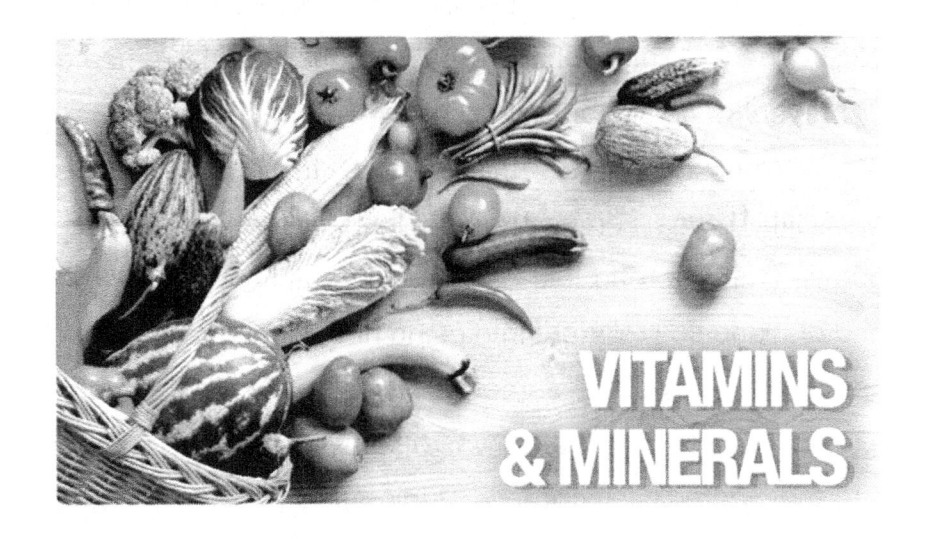

VITAMINS & MINERALS

products, however, are only available to MD's, chiropractors, licensed massage therapists and other health professionals. Having no degrees or licenses in any of those fields, I used Sarah's accounts with those companies; I was working on my own, but in her office and under her tutelage. These homeopathic remedies do not have to be prescribed by MD's, but they are not generally available over the counter.

When I went out on my own and had my own practice, I teamed up with a massage therapist and was able to establish accounts for us with Standard Process and Nutri-West. Nature's Sunshine is another company which provides good products. I believe it is a company like Avon or Amway in that you can be a distributor without having to be a health professional, but they do not make glandular extracts.

If nutrition is as foreign to you as Greek is to me, let me recommend that you acquire a book of home health remedies and/or nutritional supplements such as *Prescription for Nutritional Healing*, by Balch & Balch. Another such book is *The Practical Encyclopedia of Natural Healing,* by Mark Bricklin, editor of *Prevention* magazine, from Rodale Press.

Get a good nutritional healing reference book!

You can use these books to look up symptoms and see what supplements are recommended. Then dowse to see if the recommended supplements will benefit you or the person you are testing, and if so, then dowse to determine the amounts needed and how many times a day. Also ask if there are other supplements that would be better or should be used in addition to what you have already found. Ask if the program you are setting up is going to be the most effective way to heal the root cause and the respective symptoms of the particular situation at hand. Can you see how dowsing soon becomes such an integral part of your life that you dowse everything? Free yourself to ask, and ask, and ask. We have all the answers inside us – and/or the vibrational energy to get the answers for the person we are testing; we are all connected.

Now, if you have found that your body is asking for 1,000 mgs. of Vitamin C every 3 hours so that you can get rid of the cold that your son brought home from daycare, you might want to ask if you can **broadcast** for that Vitamin C instead of having to go out to the health food store in the snow and sleet to buy it since you feel so miserable. There is an article in the Fall 1998 *Quarterly of the American Society of*

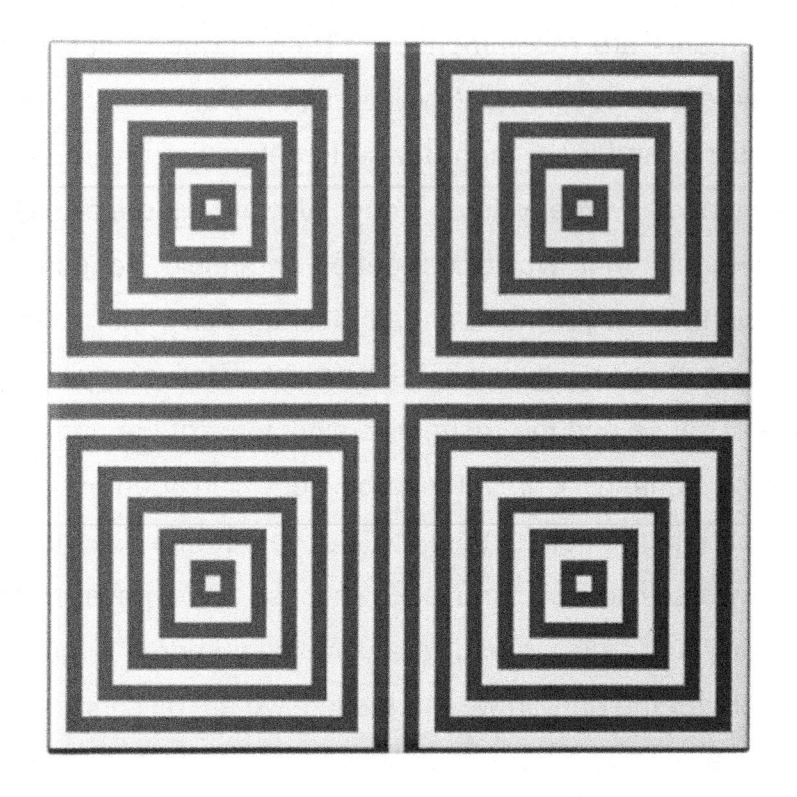

In a class I took studying learning disabilities – or better said "learning styles" – I was taught that some people have visual and audial eccentricities that make it very difficult for them to learn in traditional ways. Looking at a graphic pattern such as this before trying to read, or using a transparent overlay of a colored plastic, can transform a written page from a chaotic jumbled mess into a "normal" coherent essay for a learner who has eccentric neurons.

REMEDIES

Dowsers, by Robert Hirschfeld, entitled "Magnet Broadcasting." This article tells you how to set up a horseshoe magnet on a circle of paper and request the nutrition you need to heal your cold or root cause.

Again, this is a simple, straightforward and effective process. Ask for what you want: the Universe is here to provide our every desire.

Anne Brewer, author of THE POWER OF TWELVE, *Achieving 12-Strand DNA Consciousness* and *Breaking Free to Health,* ..., etc., writes about the efficacy of crystals and gemstones for broadcasting, combined with "Pyramid Paper" (similar to the grid pattern on the opposite page), to request and receive our desires from the Universe.

At this point I would also like to mention the book, *Spiritual Value of Gem Stones*, by Wally and Jenny Richardson and Lenora Huett. This book is very useful for healing purposes, and while its title states its spiritual or metaphysical perspective, those of you who know a lot more about stones and mineralogy than I do might find this a better reference book than a nutritional one.

The third remedy I listed above is that of "clearing." Everything, and I do mean *every thing*, is about energy. Use

BODY SPEAK

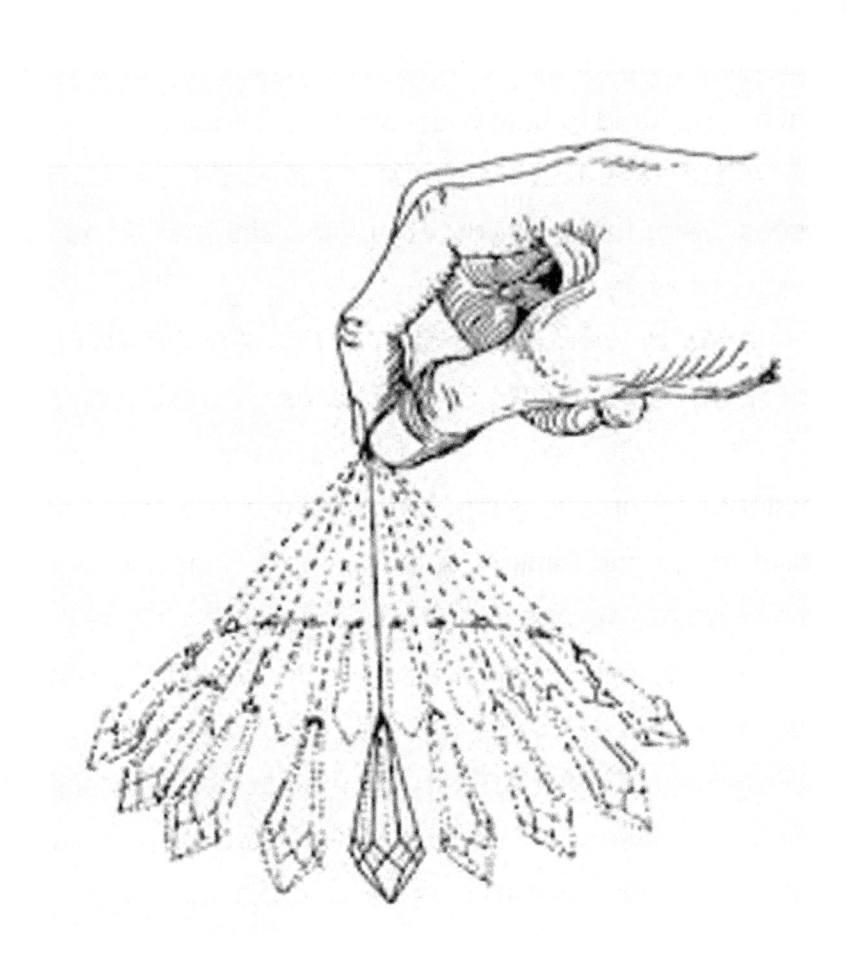

Clearing

your fingers or your pendulum to ask if you can heal yourself or the person with whom you are working by clearing the [negative] energy. When I get a positive answer to this question, I use a pendulum and swing it in a clockwise circle, rapidly, until I feel the spinning winding down - by itself - and it settles into a positive swing (for me that is away from me and back, in a straight line). I am using this method right now, every night, in order to improve my vision; I do not want to invest in glasses; besides they pinch my nose and ears.

Walt Woods, a past president of the American Society of Dowsers, used this method to heal himself of dyslexia which had plagued him his entire life. It took about two and one-half years of clearing or asking for a healing of his DNA, but it definitely worked. I know because I edited his "President's Comments" for the ASD Quarterly several years – and there was almost nothing to edit. I love the way this works! And ask how long it will take to clear. I'm not suggesting it will take years to clear or change or heal a condition! Dowse it! Ask to heal quickly!

BODY SPEAK

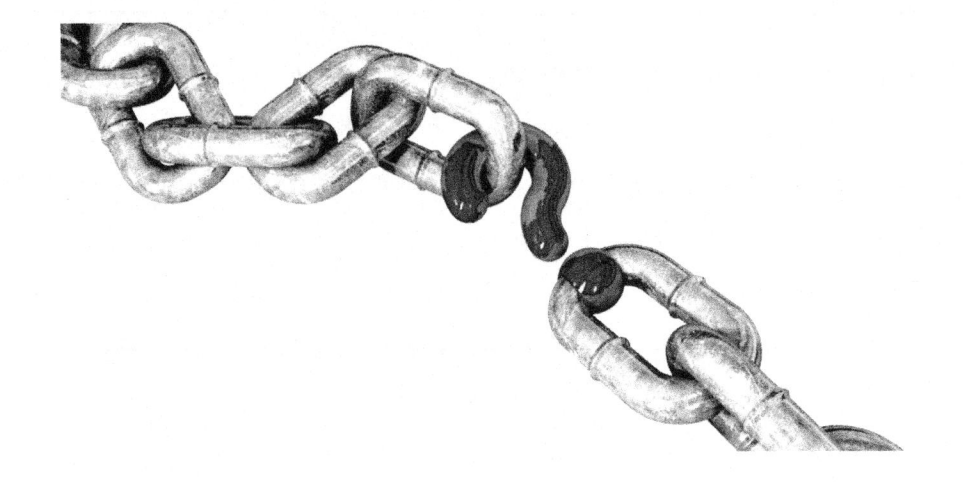

Missing Link

CHAPTER FIVE
BLOOD TYPE DIET

I have only skimmed the surface of the methods and possibilities of healing and transformation that are available to us now. For you to have been interested in *Body Speak* to begin with tells me that you have knowledge of therapies or processes that you can use to heal yourself. The miracle for me was learning how to muscle test and dowse so that I could link the symptom with the "cure." My intention in writing this book is just that: to give you the missing link – as it was given to me. There are many links, though.

And wait! I am not done with nutrition and diet yet! I must make a big side track here, Since I wrote this so many years ago, I have discovered another important reason for how and why my vegetarian pregnancy went so well:

Different blood types process and digest foods differently. Many years after I became a vegetarian and had such a wonderful, healthy pregnancy, and a wonderful, healthy child, I discovered the blood type diet - and with that

Beans and Legumes

Blood Type	Highly Beneficial	Neutral	Avoid
O	Adzuki black-eyed peas	black bean cannellini bean fava bean garbanzo bean green/string beans jicama lima mung bean / sprouts Northern pea (green / pod / snow) soybean	kidney bean lentil (domestic / green / red) navy bean pinto Tamarind
A	Adzuki beans black beans black-eyed peas fava green / string / snap beans lentil (domestic / green / red) pinto beans soybean	cannellini bean jicama mung bean / sprouts Northern pea (green/pod / snow) white bean	garbanzo kidney bean lima navy bean Tamarind
B	kidney lima navy	cannellini fava green / string / snap jicama Northern pea (green / pod / snow) tamarind white	Adzuki black black-eyed pea garbanzo lentil (domestic / green / red) mung pinto soybean
AB	green lentil navy pinto soybean	cannellini green / string / snap jicama lentil (domestic / red) Northern pea (green / pod / snow) tamarind white	Adzuki black black-eyed pea fava garbanzo kidney lima mung bean / sprouts

discovery the information that a vegetarian diet is the best for those with A type blood! Perfect for me since I am A+. On the opposite page is an example chart for the food group of beans and legumes, showing the three categories: "highly beneficial," "neutral," and "avoid," for each of the different blood types – and the beans and legumes that fall into those categories. I chose this example because I have heard so many Americans say, "I don't eat beans; they give me gas." You probably *will* have gas if you eat beans that you should 'avoid.' I have found it to be true! Beans are an important part of my vegetarian diet. I don't want to have indigestion all the time!

Speaking very generally: O blood type needs a high protein / low carbohydrate diet which includes red meat. A-type blood people needs lot of carbohydrates, but low fat: no meat, very little animal protein. B-type blood can tolerate some dairy; AB is a combination of A-type and B-type.

The differences in how people with different blood types digest their food were discovered by Dr. James D'Adamo, a naturopath, who began his practice in the 1970's, and went on to refine his discovery to include sub-types in the different blood types. For example, my major or primary blood

BODY SPEAK

BLOOD TYPES of BABY

	\multicolumn{4}{c}{Father's blood type}
Mother's blood type	A	B	AB	O
A	A, O	A, B, AB, O	A, B, AB	A, O
B	A, B, AB, O	B, O	A, B, AB	B, O
AB	A, B, AB	A, B, AB	A, B, AB	A, B
O	A, O	B, O	A, B	O

type is A. My subgroup is B. I found this out when I went to The D'Adamo Institute in Portsmouth, New Hampshire.

My daughter is also A+, but her sub-type is O. If you knew us at all well, I think you would understand. O blood types need meat – red meat. I think of them as having more aggressive personalities and physical natures. My daughter is much more ambitious than I am; she's an independent, hard-working mother AND business woman! She has married an Indian, a Hindu family, and her mother-in-law (B blood type) is a strict lacto-vegetarian, but not 'ovo.' Milk is okay, but not eggs! My daughter and her husband, whose blood type is O, are quite content with his mother's cooking at home - it's delicious and healthy - but when they eat out, they usually add meat. It seems to work well.

Dr. James D'Adamo passed away in 2013, but his work is being continued through multidisciplinary therapies including acupuncture, weight loss, chiropractic, iridology, and others, as well as the nutritional therapy. Dr. James D'Adamo's second book: *Just An Ounce of PREVENTION ... Is Worth A Pound of CURE*, covers his last research of the subgroup blood types and is fascinating and informative.

BODY SPEAK

You are perfect exactly the way you are.

Werner Erhard

BLOOD TYPE DIET

Dr. Peter D'Adamo, the son of Dr. James D'Adamo, also a naturopath, has his own practice and has continued the blood type diet, but he has gone a different route and instead of blood-type subgroups, he is using genotypes for making more specific therapies for patients. His first book, *Eat Right 4 Your Type*, which has been expanded in subsequent books, states the basic differences in blood types and lists foods by "Highly Beneficial," "Neutral," and "Avoid" and for the different blood types. Just using the charts has made a big difference for me, with little effort: I have no trouble substituting grapefruit for oranges, for example.

I found this quote on Dr. Peter's website and I think it's very interesting that Japan is so invested in this diet.

> What are your thoughts on the level of devotion to blood type in Japanese society? They market soft drinks and condoms according to blood type! Do you think Americans will ever go so far?

Most Americans have no idea of their personal blood type; doctors don't tell us nowadays; it is not on our birth certificates or in our medical files. If you would like to know your blood type without having to pay a big laboratory fee,

BODY SPEAK

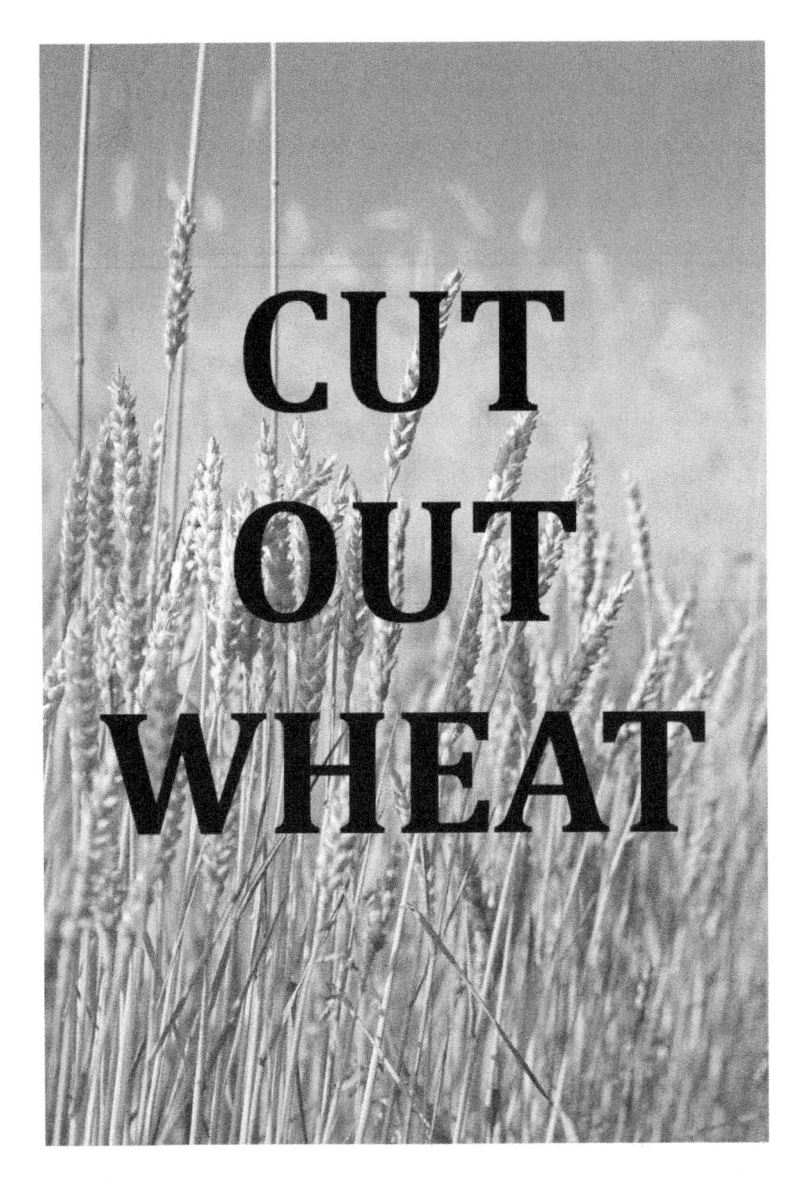

CUT OUT WHEAT

I'm sorry!

order the kit from www.4yourtype.com and for $9.95 per kit, and about five minutes, once you receive the kit, you will know your blood type!

One "universal" truth from this blood type diet is: WHEAT is NOT GOOD for ANY BODY! Especially as it has been genetically modified, *in this country*; and the chemicals that are used, *in this country*, to process it. Europe and Australia, in particular, have banned the chemicals we use to process our wheat.

My experience following the blood type diet has been profound. I can't help but think this is a major part of being healthy and having a strong immune system. Eat what is best for you, because you are what you eat.

The whole point of this book is to show you ways you can maintain your health, and heal if you have problems. I don't want to suffer. I don't want anyone else to suffer! So let's ask the right questions and listen to our bodies speak.

BODY SPEAK

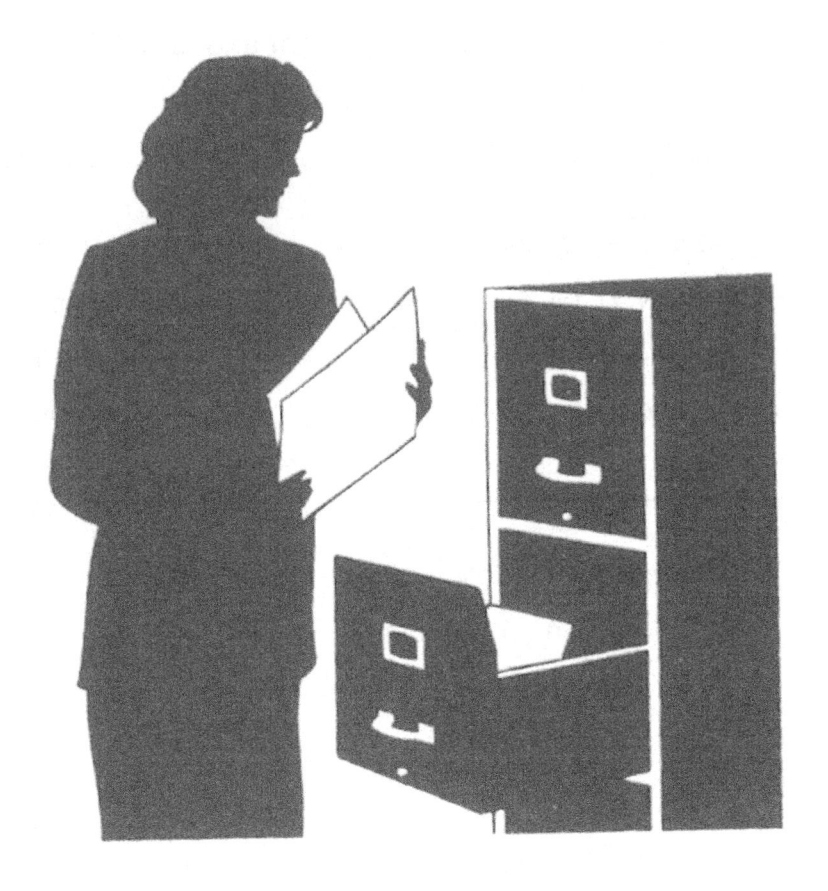

What will we find filed away in our minds?

CHAPTER SIX

NEURO-EMOTIONAL RELEASING

Nutrition is not always the answer to a person's problems. Let us come back from the boulevard of diet and supplements and look at some other suggestions for problems, symptoms and root causes.

If you were testing someone for a root cause of a symptom and the Emotional point blew, I said to see this Chapter – so here we are. This chapter could easily be a book in itself, and There ARE books out there. And very effective therapies: The Emotion Code is one. But right now, at this time, I give you these charts to use for testing the emotional body, and for discovering thought forms that have gotten stuck in the emotional body and created illness. I will also show you the process of releasing and clearing memories and trauma so that healing and recovery can take place.

When I learned "NER" from Sarah Meredith in 1992, she had recently channeled this technique and its accompanying charts and particularities. NER covers much more than the emotional body, but I have simplified this system a great deal – partly because I never did completely understand Sarah's process and more because I learned

BODY SPEAK

Neuro-Emotional Releasing

Pineal	Speechless, blind, dumb, tongue-tied, unsociable, purposeless, powerless, unconcerned, perception twisted, faulty perception, can't 'see,' foggy awareness, deaf, empty, use your innate.
Hypothalamus Thymus Pituitary	Not desirable, not needed, not wanted, failure, hunger, deprived, thirst, not centered, not important, not appreciated, troubled, difficult, hard, too much responsibility, trying, imposed upon, forgetful, neglected, use your innate
Parotid Thyroid Heart	Unhappy, grouchy, argumentative, disappointed, pain, belligerent, stubborn, non-thinking, non-emotive, depleted, suppressed, sluggish memory, vivid dreaming, us your innate Shamed, humiliated, fearful, terror, not respected, unworthy, defensive, stupid, made a fool of, put down, muddled instability, paranoia, muddled thinking, emotional instability, up and down, can't figure it out
Parathyroid Adrenals Small Intestine	Frightfully overjoyed, abnormal (inappropriate) laughing, lack of emotion, rapid mannerisms, insecure, bitter, unloved, forgotten, broken-hearted, defeated, sour, disgusted, rapid speech, selfish, pressured, compelled, not giving, deceitful, unfriendly
Ovaries Uterus Prostate Testicles	Anxious, irritated, frustrated, concerned, jealous, repressed, suppressed, paranoid, used, let down, troubled, fretful, vulnerable, abandoned, deserted, absent mindedness, insecurity, lost profoundly deep unreturned love, unappreciated, forced, obligated Worried, misunderstood, dirty, not fruitful, not productive, wrong, misjudged, not responsive, frigid, not fulfilled, dishonorable, unrecognized, unthinking, thoughtless, not affectionate, liar
Eye	Overwhelmed, over-taxed, shattered, forsaken, abandoned, clingy, not willing to know (Past, Present, Future), not willing to see (Past, Present, Future), longing, yearning, not motivated, not successful
Ear	Unsupportive, can't help, guilty, repulsive, abhorrent, vindictive, not helpful, irresponsible, not interested, bored, not willing to listen, heard something hurtful, closing out the world, not willing to hear your inner voice, use your innate

about Spiritual Response Therapy which covers a great deal more than NER does. What I am presenting here is only the *emotional body* part of NER. If while using NER you find that you need to probe more deeply, or are discovering problems in bodies other than the emotional one, see Chapter 7 so that you can connect with Spiritual Response Therapy and/or find an Emotion Code practitioner!! Dowse what the best therapy is and then continue with the more physical problems.

Don't immediately sell Neuro Emotional Releasing short, however. I feel strongly that NER is a very efficient and effective tool for clearing emotional causes of illness. If we really are 90% emotions, how can any of us escape the nicks and bungs that occur in our daily lives?

The opposite and reverse pages of this page are charts that you can use to test with. What I usually do is to put my probe hand palm down on the first chart and ask, "Does this chart contain the root cause of (your client)'s symptom?" And then I ask the person to pull, or I use my own fingers or a pendulum if I am doing a remote viewing. If the answer is no, I go the next chart and ask. (You can work on your own emotional problems, but make sure that you are as focused

BODY SPEAK

Neuro-Emotional Releasing

Stomach	Disgust, low self-esteem, expanded importance of self, obsession, egotistic despair, nervous, lives through others, over concern, hopelessness, lack of control over events, harsh
Spleen	Over sympathetic to another, unreliable, repulsive, disgusted, discontent, impatient, nauseated, resentful, not submissive, rebellious, upset, not courageous, insignificant, worthless
Pancreas	Useless, betrayed, rejected, sorrow, pity, not accepted, given to pint of exhaustion, can't take any more, giving up, not wanting to repair or rebuild, depleted, empty, rejecting life, hard to admit or accept, cutting use your innate
Left Lung	Grief for others, grief for self, cloudy thinking, sadness, yearning, anguish, drying, compelled to neatness, defensive, dogmatically positioned, depressed, criticized, recluse
Right Lung Large Intestine	Out of sorts, unfriendly, exasperated, forlorn, lonely, left out, envy, crying, doubt, cut off, barrier, disunited, incomprehensible, at wits' end, lost use your innate
Kidney	Fear, miffed, pissed out, dread, bad memory, paralyzed will, contemplate, timid, inefficient, wishy-washy, intolerant, disloyal, ashamed, at fault, aggressive, use your innate
Bladder Urinary Tract	Hate, revolting, anger, injustice, futile, weary, tired, wasted, embarrassed, shy, in vain, impossible, panful to release, holding on, shame, getting even, let go, letting go, can't let go, whatever will be will be
Gall Bladder	Resentment, anger, galled, stubborn, emotionally repressed, depressed, indecisive, irrationality, frustration, aggression, proud, egotistical, stuck-up, scared, decrepit, use your innate
Liver Skin	Disorganized, haughty, smug, arrogant, confused, distressed, hopeless, despair, helpless, incapable, left out hurt, uneasy, icky, unpleasant, apprehensive, creepy, squeamish, restless
Brain	Inadequate, depleted, drained, cannot, introverted, not respected, unloved, hurried, demanded upon, indecisive, stifled, blocked, pushed, rushed, agitated, not enough, pressured

as you can be on your <u>higher</u> self. It is easy to trick yourself, especially with emotional issues.)

Once you have narrowed down which of the two charts is applicable to the situation at hand, dowse which set of words and phrases is the correct one, and then narrow it down again to the particular line of words within the section. When you have the definitive line, go word-by-word or phrase-by-phrase, until you have a match – which means that your fingers will fly apart because that word or phrase will be the cause of the emotional block or trauma.

You have probably noticed the list of glands and organs in the left-hand column. I use that list mostly as an indicator of the accuracy of my dowsing. Sometimes the section that I find the word or thought in has the exact organ listed in the left-hand column, across from the words. Other times, I find that my higher self, or the person's higher self that I am testing, has chosen a spot that is actually the root cause of a symptom I have not even been asking about and is more problematical to me or the other person than the one I have been dowsing for. You may already know how our brains protect themselves, and how a symptom may be covering up

BODY SPEAK

Chakra	Color	Archangel
1. Root	Red	**Kamiel** Light, Power, Energy
2. Pelvic	Orange	**Zadkiel** Materialization, Creative Visualization
3. Solar Plexus	Yellow	**Zophkiel** Art, Beauty, Perfection, Balance
4. Heart	Green	**Auriel** Nature, Compassion
5. Throat	Blue	**Gabriel** Sound, Vibration, Communication
6. Brow	Indigo	**Michael** Protection, Truth
7. Crown	Violet	**Raphael** Healing, Love

from *Power of Twelve*
and *Spiritual Value of Gems*

a much worse problem which, for some reason, we have not wanted to examine.

Once a word or phrase has been hit upon, the next step is to ask the person you are working with what that word or phrase means to them. Most times, the person will immediately identify with the word and you can see the painfully emotional connection in their face or answer. If there is no apparent connection or response from the word, ask them to give you a definition of that word. It is not unusual for a person to have the wrong definition of a word "programmed" into their brain. And it often follows that the person has emotional trauma from miscommunication because of the incorrect definition – OR that the incorrect definition was created to mask a trauma related to the CORRECT definition!

It is helpful to have a dictionary to refer to when working with NER. Since the problems all stem from words and their real or perceived definitions, it is good to keep in touch with "reality." And a good dictionary to have is Webster's New World Dictionary for Young Readers since many of these thought forms are created when we are young.

There is no time like the present.

What a gift!

See what memories come up for the person when you say the word or phrase to them.

Ask them to think of a memory related to the word or phrase that came before that one.

Ask them to think of the FIRST TIME the word or phrase produced a bad memory or experience.

Ask if they are ready to clear the memories. If so, clear. If not, ask for memories from previous lives, or before the "first time" they told you. When the person is ready to clear, your fingers will hold very firm.

To clear: ask the person to hold their breath while you run your probe hand up and then down the spine (not quite touching it) once. Then ask the person to breathe in while you "sweep" the spine down; and then to breathe out while you sweep your hand up the spine. And it's done.

You should explain to the person that the memory will remain with them, but the emotional charge will be greatly reduced. Also warn the person that this "clearing" is only as effective as their resolve not to recreate the memory by dwelling on it or bringing it again to mind.

This process is fast and efficient, not to mention it really works.

BODY SPEAK

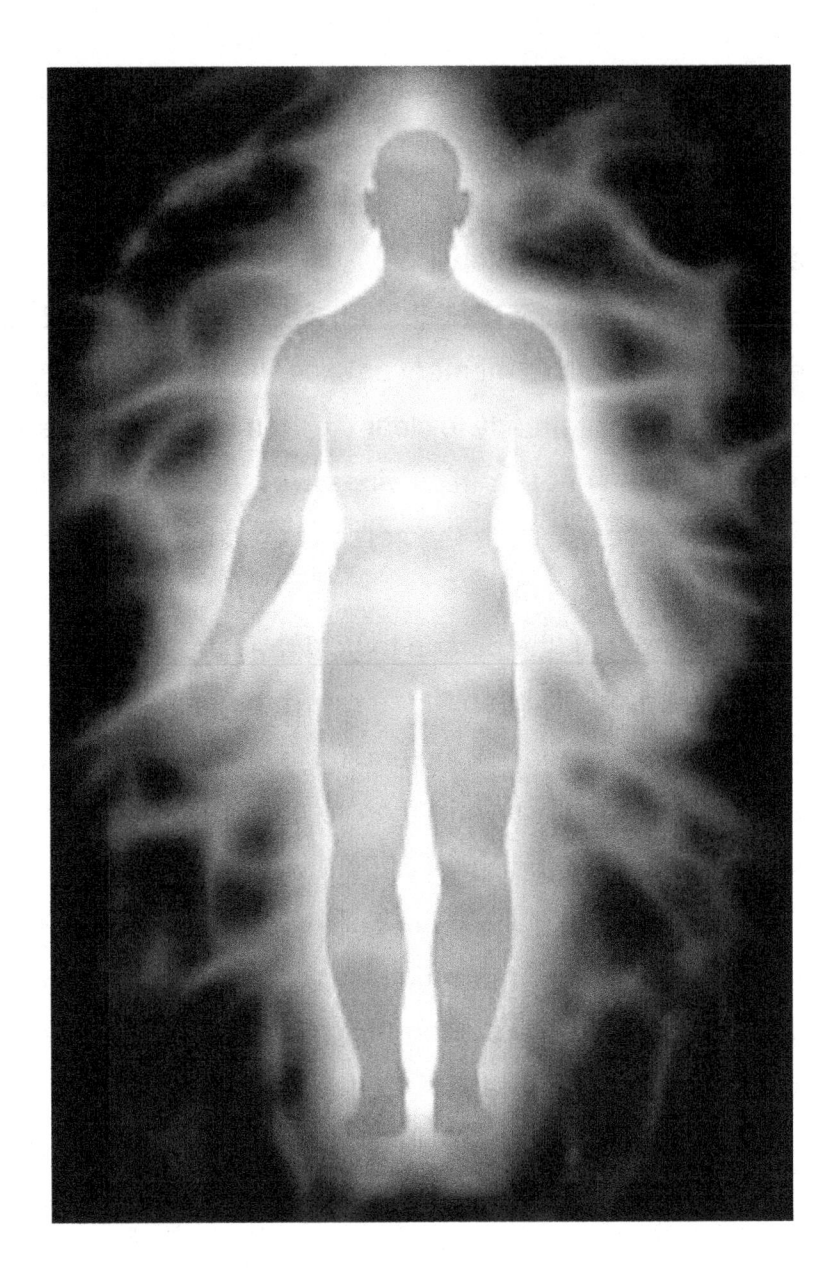

CHAPTER SEVEN

SPIRITUAL RESPONSE THERAPY

If you went through all the physical body points, both primary and secondary, AND the emotional point on the brow and STILL did not get a response, the SPIRITUAL BODIES point probably will oblige! And I hope you won't be disappointed that at this POINT I am going to recommend you to Spiritual Response Therapy. Dowse it, of course!

Spiritual Response Association
1880 Barnes Blvd. SW, B1
Tumwater, WA 98512
web site: www.spiritualresponse.com
Check the website and/or call for consulting hours.
(360) 413-7881

I took a class in Spiritual Response Therapy in 1995, from Nina Brown in Oakland, California, and in 2005, I did a review and then took Advanced SRT. I never became a teacher of SRT, but I did use it – A LOT. This body of knowledge and its associated techniques for clearing and healing is extensive and profound. Until we all reach our spiritual body stage of evolution, however, we do have to deal with our earthsuits and try to keep them as clean, pressed and lint free as possible!

YOU BECOME WHAT YOU THINK.

Jesus Christ
Napoleon Hill
Wayne Dyer
Norman Vincent Peale
Deepak Chopra, et al.

SPIRITUAL RESPONSE THERAPY

I can recommend the Spiritual Response Association and its Therapy to anyone who truly wishes to heal and transform his or her life. I had valuable experience with SRT, and the Association has continued to develop Dr. Robert Detzler's therapy since he made his transition.

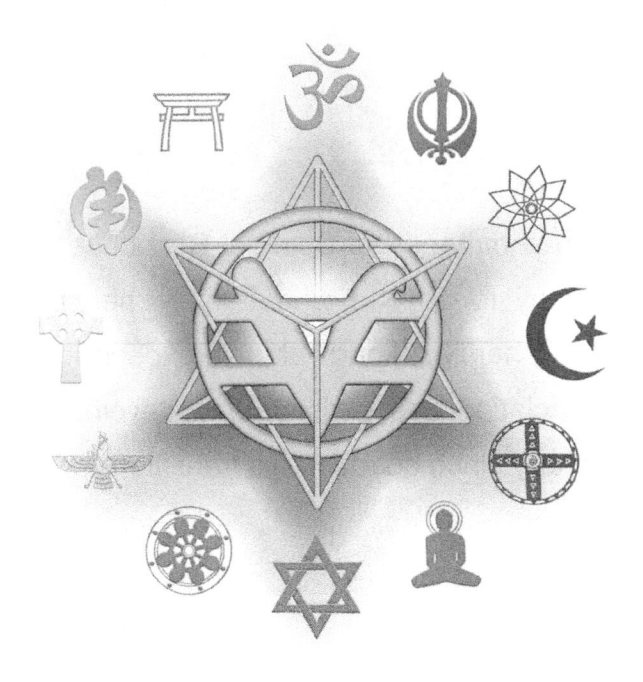

A New Thought "logo"
We are all ONE – ALL INCLUSIVE!

CHAPTER EIGHT

Moving Higher with NEW THOUGHT

It's hard to believe that I first wrote Body Speak in 1998, more than 20 years ago. I met my first spiritual teacher, Unity minister Rev. Edwene Gaines, nine years before that, in 1989. Her ministry is prosperity; she made a covenant with God to be 100% personally responsible for raising the prosperity/abundance consciousness of this planet. True prosperity includes, of course, perfect health.

I grew up attending a Presbyterian church, the logical choice of an English-Scottish mother and English-German father, living in the South. My mother was also a health food aficionado, reading everything written by Adele Davis, and following her advice to a great extent. I'm grateful for the good food and nutritional principles of "health food," even though I can't say the same for the church … I left the church, at least in my mind and spirit, when my dad died in 1959. I couldn't believe God would take him away, leaving me stuck with my mother who was still angry at me for not being a male to carry on the family name. Those were my erroneous beliefs then. About God.

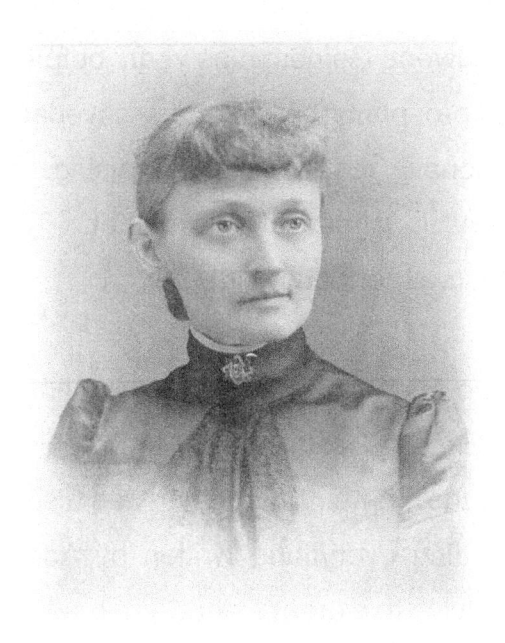

Emma Curtis Hopkins
"The Teacher of Teachers"
of New Thought

NEW THOUGHT

The interest in health food stuck, however, even though I rebelled against it, as any self-respecting teenager would do. I returned to it as soon as I was on my own and in charge of my own meals after college, however!

Then, when I learned to dowse and muscle test in 1992, the three things of nutrition, spirituality, and dowsing came together and brought me to the point of writing *Body Speak* in 1998. I had the motivation of presenting it at a Dowsers' conference in 1999, in Houston, and I got it done. Twenty years can't go by, however, without some change; and there has been considerable.

Slowly, over the years, I got more and more involved in the spiritual community I was introduced to when I heard Edwene at her prosperity seminar. My studies became more intellectual, then spiritual, and while I do my best to care for my physical body with nutrition, and dowsing for root causes of symptoms, I have turned more and more to the mystical and spiritual studies for my REAL LIFE. We are here to learn and grown – and to REALIZE the PERFECT BEINGS that we are. We are expressions of Divine Mind.

BODY SPEAK

OMNIPRESENT

OMNISCIENT

OMNIPRESENT

God

NEW THOUGHT

I have spent more and more time focusing on spiritual studies. The belief that I have come to through my studies and experiences in New Thought and its principles (this is not a religion) is that there is One Presence, that is Omnipresent, Omniscient and Omnipotent, and that that Presence is GOOD. 'New Thought' means just that: choose new thoughts of good, positivity; raise your consciousness and change your life. I believe this is Truth.

Coming to the end of my book, and looking out to what may lie ahead, anticipation and excitement overwhelm me. What a glorious time we live in: on the edge of timelessness and oneness with the Universe! Knowing that I cannot even imagine what is to come, I wait – without much patience – and I reach out for your hand so we can fly together. Our divine purpose and responsibilities are to have as much fun as we can possibly have – and share it. And truly, there is no time like the present. What a gift!

KNOW:

> If you want to change your life, change your mind.
> You are loved unconditionally, always.
> There is always enough.

BODY SPEAK

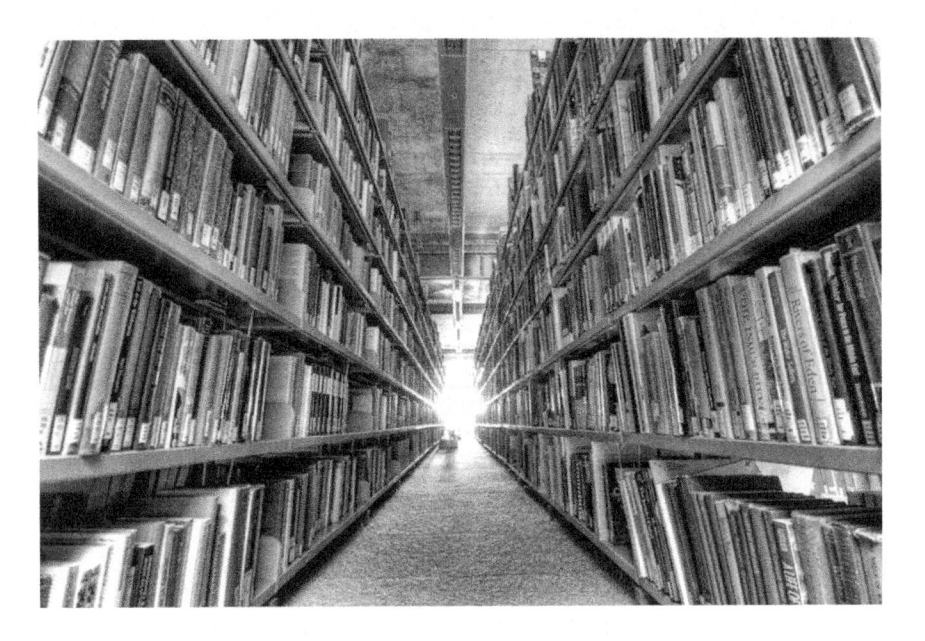

We have endless resources
and infinite potential!

BIBLIOGRAPHY

Balch, James F. and Balch, Phyllis A. *Prescription for Nutritional Healing: A Practical A-Z Reference to Drug-free Remedies Using Vitamins, Minerals, Herbs and Food Supplements and Prescription for Nutritional Healing A-To-Z Guide to Supplements: A Handy Resource to Today's Most Effective Nutritional Supplements.* Paperback.

Brewer, Anne. *The Power of Twelve, 12-Strand DNA Consciousness.* Hygiene, Colorado: Sunshine Press Publications, Inc., 1998.

Bricklin, Mark. *The Practical Encyclopedia of Natural Healing.* Emmaus, Pennsylvania: Rodale Press, Inc. 1976.

Clark, Linda. *The Ancient Art of Color Therapy.* New York.

D'Adamo, James, with Richards, Allan. *Just An Ounce of Prevention Is Worth a Pound of Cure.* Carlsbad, California: Hay House, Inc., 2010.

D'Adamo, Peter, with Whitney, Catherine. *Eat Right 4 Your Type.* New York: G. P. Putnam's Sons, 1996; New York: New American Library, 2016.

Davis, Adelle. *Let's Cook It Right*; *Let's Eat Right To Keep Fit*; and *Let's Get Well.* New York: Harcourt, Brace Jovanovich, 1970; 1970; and 1965, respectively.

Detzler, Robert E. *The Freedom Path: Your Mind Net To Clear Your Soul Records.* Redmond, Washington.

Hopkins, Emma Curtis. *High Mysticism* and *Scientific Christian Mental Practice.* Marina del Rey, California: DeVorss & Co. (originally published by High Watch Society, Cornwall Bridge, Connecticut.)

Hay, Louise L. *Heal Your Body*; and *You Can Heal Your Life.* Carson, California: Hay House, Inc., 1988, and 1984.

Lacy, Louise. *Lunaception: A Feminine Odyssey Into Fertility And Contraception.* Warner Books, 1976.

Lee, John R. *Natural Progesterone.* 1955 and later.

Lee, John R. and Hopkins, Virginia L. *Natural Progesterone: What Your Doctor May Not Tell You About Menopause.* 1996.

Myss, Caroline. *Why People Don't Heal and How They Can*; and *Anatomy of the Spirit.* New York: Harmony Books, 1996; and 1988.

Myss, Caroline and Shealy, Norman C. *The Creation of Health.* New York: Harmony Books, 1997.

Nelson, Bradley. *The Emotion Code* (expanded and revised edition). New York: St. Martin's Press, 2019.

Peale, Norman Vincent. *Stay Alive All Your Life*; and *The Power of Positive Thinking.* Pawling, New York: Peale Center for Christian Living, 1957; and 1952.

BIBLIOGRAPHY

Ponder, Catherine. *Open Your Mind To Receive*. Marina del Rey, California: DeVorss & Co., 1983.

Richardson, Wally, and Richardson, Jenny, and Huett, Lenora. *The Spiritual Value of Gem Stones*. Marina del Rey, California: DeVorss & Co., 1988.

Weil, Andrew. *8 Weeks To Optimum Health* (video), and *Chocolate To Morphine*. New York: Houghton Mifflin, 1983.

Weil, Andrew. *Common Illnesses*. New York: Ivy Books, 1997.

Woods, Walter. *Letter To Robin*. Self-published. Danville, Vermont: available from American Society of Dowsers Bookstore and online.

LOOK UP!

Made in the USA
Columbia, SC
16 March 2025